# THE POCKET GUIDE TO THERAPY

STEPHEN WEATHERHEAD & GRAEME FLAHERTY-JONES

# THE POCKET GUIDE TO THERAPY

## A 'HOW TO' OF THE CORE MODELS

SAGE

Los Angeles | London | New Delhi
Singapore | Washington DC

First published 2012



SAGE Publications Ltd
1 Oliver's Yard
55 City Road
London EC1Y 1SP

SAGE Publications Inc.
2455 Teller Road
Thousand Oaks, California 91320

SAGE Publications India Pvt Ltd
B 1/I 1 Mohan Cooperative Industrial Area
Mathura Road, Post Bag 7
New Delhi 110 044

SAGE Publications Asia-Pacific Pte Ltd
33 Pekin Street #02-01
Far East Square
Singapore 048763

**Library of Congress Control Number: 2011924685**

**British Library Cataloguing in Publication data**

A catalogue record for this book is available from the British Library

ISBN 978-0-85702-492-3
ISBN 978-0-85702-493-0 (pbk)

Typeset by C&M Digitals (P) Ltd, Chennai, India
Printed and bound by CPI Group (UK) Ltd, Croydon, CRO 4YY
Printed on paper from sustainable resources

For Claire and Elliott
The voice of reason and reason for being.

*G.M.F-J.*

For Claire and Euan (my world), Dad (my inspiration),
and John Allen (The Pioneer of Fun)

*S.J.W.*

# CONTENTS

# ABOUT THE EDITORS

**Stephen Weatherhead** qualified as a Clinical Psychologist in 2008. Since then he has specialised in brain injury within the NHS, and private practice. Stephen has just taken up a full-time position with Lancaster University and Lancashire Care NHS Foundation Trust as a Lecturer in Health Research and Clinical Tutor, with the DClinPsy course. His publications and research reflect his therapeutic interests in neuropsychology, narrative and systemic therapies, qualitative approaches, cultural issues, and evidencing outcomes. Stephen thinks therapy is as much an art as it is a science, and that part of the role of the therapist is to make it accessible. That's why he aimed to write this book in a way that demystifies the theory and application of therapy for the newcomer. www.neurofamilymatters.co.uk

**Graeme Flaherty-Jones** is a Specialist Clinical Psychologist based across Middlesbrough, Redcar and Cleveland, where he has the pleasure of working with older people within Tees, Esk and Wear Valleys/NHS Foundation Trust. Outside of the NHS he also has a private practice called Clarity Psychology. Aside from his clinical work Graeme enjoys contributing to publications on behalf of his professional body, the British Psychological Society, and providing teaching on the doctorate course in Clinical Psychology at Teesside University. An overarching ethos to all aspects of his professional work is a desire to make psychological theory accessible so that it may benefit others. He hopes that this ethos will come across in the pages of this book which offers an introduction to the exciting world of therapy.
www.claritypsychology.com

# ABOUT THE AUTHORS

**Phillippa Calvert** qualified as a Clinical Psychologist in 2009 from the University of Liverpool (UK). She works part-time in the NHS with adults who are experiencing severe and enduring mental health problems and those with a diagnosis of personality disorder. Phillippa also works part-time in the independent sector specialising in neuropsychology, offering psychological therapy to individuals who have been involved in serious accidents and family interventions. It was during her third year specialist placement that she participated in a Dialectic Behaviour Therapy (DBT) Skills Group and the approach had a significant impact on her. Since then she has applied the philosophy and techniques alongside other approaches such as Cognitive Analytic Therapy (CAT) and Acceptance and Commitment Therapy (ACT).

**Kara Garforth** is a Clinical Psychologist and qualified from the Lancaster Training course in 2009. She is currently employed in Pennine Care NHS Foundation Trust in Bury, Greater Manchester as part of a Secondary Care Psychological Therapies Service. Kara works with adults with severe and enduring mental health problems, conducting individual therapy and also works closely with staff in Community Mental Health Teams in a consultancy role. She is particularly interested in working with people with interpersonal difficulties and personality disorders and uses a psychodynamically informed approach to promote understanding of the impact of these difficulties on individuals' lives.

**Claire Robson** began her career in clinical psychology working in a drug and alcohol inpatient unit as an Assistant Psychologist, where she trained to use Motivational Interviewing (MI). She later completed her formal clinical psychology training at Lancaster University. She now works with adults who have moderate mental health difficulties in a primary care psychological therapies service, using an integrative approach to therapy. Claire hopes that her chapter will provide an accessible summary of MI and inspire clinicians to use an 'MI style' of interacting with clients who are ambivalent about changing their behaviours.

**Jane Toner** qualified as a Clinical Psychologist in 2008 and is a busy mum of two boys. Since qualifying as a Psychologist she has worked with looked after children. Jane now works in the independent sector, working therapeutically with young people with complex mental health and emotional needs. This work requires a lot of creative use of therapy, but also lots of consultation, teaching and training with other professionals. Jane finds this a really rewarding role. Prior to her clinical training Jane worked in the NHS as a Mental Health Nurse and CBT therapist.

**Amie Smith** is a Clinical Psychologist working across the lifespan with people with learning disabilities, their families and carers. She draws on a range of therapeutic approaches in her work, most notably systemic and psychodynamic. She puts particular value on therapists reflecting on the process of therapy, including the therapeutic relationship, and sees both of these approaches as providing frameworks to enable this reflection.

**Katie Splevins** is a journalist and Clinical Psychologist. Her passions include working cross-culturally, with specific interests in trauma and post-traumatic growth. Meditation is something Katie values enormously as part of her own life and enjoys sharing with other people.

**Fiona Syme** is a Clinical Psychologist based in the South-West of England and really enjoys her current post working with children and young people with learning difficulties and mental health issues. Outside the NHS, she has a developing private practice called 'Clarity Psychology' which she shares with Graeme Flaherty-Jones. Fiona has many clinical interests including paediatrics, eating disorders and autism. She particularly enjoy working creatively with the 'supporting system' around clients, be that families or staffing groups, to enhance clients' care. Forming strong therapeutic relationships is at the heart of her work and she prides herself on being able to meet the unique needs of her clients in a style that suits them. As a recently qualified Clinical Psychologist, Fiona is delighted to contribute to a book which seeks to bring together different types of therapy in one accessible volume.

**Sharon Twigg** started her career as a qualified counsellor and college mentor on the Wirral. She later worked as an Assistant Psychologist at Alder Hey Children's Hospital and the Walton Neurological Centre in Aintree. Sharon then continued her career by formally qualifying as a Clinical Psychologist at the University of Lancaster. She now works in the NHS and provides psychological support for children and their families on the Wirral. Sharon works part-time within paediatric liaison and part-time within the Wirral children's CAMHS service.

# ACKNOWLEDGEMENTS

There are many people who have been pivotal in bringing this book to fruition. Given the early stage we are at in our careers, it has meant them putting a tremendous amount of faith in us. We are grateful to all of you. Special thanks to: 'The Claires', who share the same name, the same commitment, and the same faith in us, and 'The Little Dudes', Elliott and Euan – all four of you keep us smiling. Our wider families, from whom we gain strength and unconditional love. Michael Carmichael, Alice Oven, Kate Wharton and Katherine Haw from SAGE, thank you for all your guidance and positivity. Tim Cate, Laura Golding, Anna Daiches and Jane Simpson, thank you for giving us the confidence to take the first strides. Steve Fuller, you are and forever will be our guru. All the co-authors, you have been brilliant, without you there would be no book, and Sally, thank you for your hawk-eye reviews.

Throughout this book you will notice that two symbols frequently appear in text boxes, which are designed to highlight key learning points for each model of therapy. The two symbols used are:

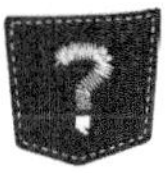

This image appears where points relate to the more philosophical/theoretical aspects of the therapeutic model being discussed.

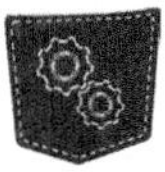

Comments where this symbol appears are akin to tutoring on therapy training courses in that they attempt to link theory and practice.

# 1 PRINCIPLES OF THERAPY

Graeme Flaherty-Jones and Stephen Weatherhead

Within this introductory chapter we will discuss what the book is, how to use it and how it can appeal to therapists at different levels of professional training. Taking a look back through time we will show how the application of therapeutic models has changed over the years. We will also introduce the models of therapy included in the book, discuss reasons for their selection, and will highlight commonalities between these models. Finally, this chapter will discuss the importance of a good therapeutic relationship and consider how therapists can develop the skills required for therapy.

So many of us have bought books in the past that we hoped would somehow (perhaps via osmosis) provide us with the skills required to 'do therapy'. Many books give a good grounding in the general principles of therapy, or provide a comprehensive overview of the theoretical underpinnings of any given therapy. Whilst this is clearly valuable, after reading them one rarely feels actually able to sit in a room and begin practising that particular model of therapy. Here we present something different. We can't promise learning through osmosis, or that you will earn your Jedi status as a master therapist by reading *The Pocket Guide to Therapy*. However, we hope that reading this book will increase your confidence and de-mystify the art of each therapeutic model.

This book does exactly what it says on the cover; it provides a clear introduction on 'how to' apply ten models of therapy that are widely used in practice. In each chapter we provide tangible examples of how the therapy models can be applied, through sample questions, snippets of worked examples, worksheets, and a detailed case study with diagrammatic formulation. We also provide text boxes to point you in the direction of further exploration should you wish to find out more, a glossary explaining the key terms (often confusing) used by practitioners/theorists of each model, and a list of references cited in the chapter.

## HOW TO USE THE POCKET GUIDE

We have designed this book so each chapter can be read in its own right as a guide to that particular model of therapy. We have tried to keep the chapters relatively short and each one has the same general format:

- *The Model* – This is a general introduction to the model of therapy and its theoretical underpinnings. These sections provide a whistle-stop tour of how the model came to be, but without delivering a full-blown history of the model.
- *Application* – Here we focus our attention to provide practical guidance on 'how to' apply the model. This is achieved through sharing techniques used in therapy and demonstrating these skills through short case extracts.
- *Case Example* – To demonstrate how the model of therapy can be applied in its entirety, we share a single case study and diagrammatic case formulation.[1]
- *Glossary* – Most models of therapy have their own unique terms that can sometimes feel like a foreign language. Whilst each chapter tries to avoid overuse of such language, a glossary of the key terms used within the therapeutic model is presented at the end of each chapter with 'plain English' definitions.
- *Worksheets* – At the end of each chapter, four worksheets are provided to help with applying the model in practice. You will find that these are outlined in grey shading to make them easy to locate for quick reference.

### Warning!

Reading the various chapters of this book will sadly not lead to a qualification in the particular model of therapy. Instead, we hope the chapters provide a taster of what to expect from each model of therapy, which may in turn lead you to consider further training. It is this further training that can provide the development of key skills and ultimately lead you to becoming professionally qualified in a particular model of therapy. Where possible we have tried to provide signposting to additional reading and useful resources that can help facilitate this developmental process.

## THERAPY: THEN AND NOW

Social interaction has been at the very core of our being, for as long as we have been on this earth (Mithen, 1996). We don't know exactly when these social skills were used to help each other in a therapeutic way. One widely accepted view is that what we commonly refer to as 'therapy' emerged in the latter part of the nineteenth century with the work of Sigmund Freud. In developing his psychoanalytic theory, Freud demonstrated how a conceptual understanding of the human mind might be used to bring about benefit for others in the context of therapy.

As the founding father of therapy, Freud forged a path for the development of many different theoretical models. We cover ten models in this book, all of which come under the umbrella of therapy. Without providing an exhaustive history of terminology it's probably fair to say that the most common terms for talking approaches to overcoming problems are 'therapy', 'counselling', and 'psychotherapy'. Although we use the term 'therapy' in this book, we remain mindful of the idiosyncratic differences that exist under each heading (e.g. historical roots, models of training and elements of practice), whilst acknowledging that:

> Psychotherapy, like counselling, is fundamentally talking-based therapy resting on psychological contact, theories and techniques.
>
> (Palmer, 2000: 6)

Substantial developments have occurred in the therapy field over the last century, involving a shift in both the breadth and acceptance of theoretical models. Therapists often used to operate solely within their own theoretical frameworks and exchanged insults towards alternative approaches; thankfully that conflict is less prominent these days (Norcross and Newman, 2003). While therapists may still choose to work from a single theoretical orientation, the present era has seen greater tolerance for the diversity of therapy, and some amalgamation of different models.

As theoretical divisions have become less prominent and therapy has developed into an increasingly profession-centred health practice (House, 2003), there has been a boom in new and assimilated models of therapy (e.g. cognitive analytic therapy). This recent expansion in therapeutic models can perplex even the most experienced therapist when considering which approach to work with in practice. At any stage in our career, the array of therapies out there can be overwhelming when setting out to develop a core set of skills.

We have selected ten of the most widely used therapeutic models in modern practice. In choosing ten models to form the *Pocket Guide*, certain modalities are inevitably omitted; for example, behavioural therapy is left out in place of models that integrate the approach, such as cognitive behavioural therapy and dialectical behavioural therapy. Similarly, mentalisation has not been included because it's more widely incorporated into other psychodynamic therapies. The list goes on (e.g. eye movement desensitisation and reprocessing – EMDR), and this is discussed in more detail at the end of the final chapter.

The models of therapy covered have been selected for their broad use across professional disciplines, where many are not specific to any one group of therapists. We therefore offer a starting point for all trainee and newly qualified therapists to consider the type of therapy that connects with their own interests and values. By presenting an accessible guide to the core components of each therapeutic model, we hope this book will serve as a foundation on which to develop further skills

## FORMULATION

In the context of counselling and psychotherapy, formulation refers to the use of theoretical models to reach an understanding of the problem, and can be used to inform the process of therapy. In recent times, formulation has received increasing attention within the counselling and psychotherapy field (Johnstone and Dallos, 2006). Some therapeutic models (e.g. cognitive behavioural therapy) use formulation as an integral part of the approach, and as such formulation is covered in detail within the application section of the chapter. For other therapeutic models (e.g. mindfulness) formulation is not typically used as part of therapy, but may still serve as a useful tool to inform the therapist's thinking and practice. By integrating formulation into all of the case studies, we hope to demonstrate that, above all, formulations should be meaningful to the person and therapist regardless of the theoretical model.

There is no right or wrong way of constructing a formulation, and there is no set time to begin this process in therapy. Some therapists like to start building a formulation from the notes they have gathered during the initial assessment phase of therapy, while others prefer to let the person reach their own formulation when it feels right for them. When considering how to use formulation in your practice, it can be useful to hold in mind some of these questions:

- Who will be involved in helping to construct the formulation (person in therapy, therapist, family)?
- What factors (past or present) impact on the person's difficulties and how those difficulties are managed?
- How will the formulation be used to work with the person and problem in therapy?

- What qualities or features of the person and their life can be used to overcome the problem?
- Is it helpful for the person to have explicit awareness of the formulation, or should it be used to guide the therapist's course of action?
- How might the therapist's own values, motives, assumptions and opinions impact on the formulation?
- How might aspects of the formulation impact on the therapeutic relationship?
- When would be a good time to review the formulation and amend it if necessary?

Answers to the above questions will differ for each person who accesses therapy. Formulations and therapeutic interventions should therefore be sensitive to the person and be regularly reviewed to check that they accurately take account of people's ever-changing circumstances.

## MODELS OF THERAPY: INTEGRATIVE, PURIST, AND WHERE THE BOUNDARIES BLUR

Each chapter presents a distinct model of therapy, along with some of the techniques and skills which make up that particular model. To keep the chapters focused and assist in getting to grips with the core techniques of each model, we have deliberately avoided making overt reference to other therapies within each chapter. However, as we discussed at the beginning of this chapter, recent developments in the therapy field have led to a degree of overlap between certain models.

Some therapies come from very different philosophical and historical backgrounds, which results in very different practices. However, others share common ground. Understanding these overlaps can facilitate an appreciation that developing certain skills within one particular model can sometimes provide a transferable set of skills for practising other models. Also, understanding areas of overlap advances our awareness of how to integrate different models of therapy. Developing this skill can enable therapists to eclectically tailor therapy to meet the needs of each person, should they wish to do so.

It can also be useful to think of therapeutic models as sitting along a loose continuum from scientific/positivist perspectives (such as cognitive behavioural therapy), through humanist therapies (such as person-centred counselling) and constructivist and constructionist approaches (such as narrative therapy), to the more spiritual approaches (such as mindfulness therapy).

There is no 'right way' of doing any therapy, and there are countless ways in which the many different models can be integrated. Even when thinking about what that integration may look like, therapists may choose to:

- Learn about one model of therapy and practice within this one model (purist approach).
- Learn about numerous models of therapy and apply each model separately, depending on suitability of the person accessing therapy.
- Learn multiple models of therapy and draw on aspects of each model to create an individualised therapeutic approach.

When thinking about integrating two or more models, it can be useful to think about the shared and contrasting aspects of each. Again, there is no right response to that awareness. Some people would argue that it is useful to integrate models that at the very least have a shared philosophical foundation. Others may argue that using models that are more distinct from each other allows one therapeutic model to fill the gaps in the other. Figure 1.1 may be a useful starting point for considering how the different models sit in relation to each other.

If you are going to take a purist approach (i.e. work from a single model of therapy), then there are many ways to learn about and apply each of them. When exploring this, you will constantly come across the term 'evidence-based practice' (EBP) in relation to showing that an approach can have good outcomes. Outcomes evaluation is discussed in detail in the final chapter, but by way of a foreword, EBP has been defined as:

> The integration of the best available research with clinical expertise in the context of patient characteristics, culture, and preferences.
>
> (APA, 2005: 1)

The topic of EBP has become a dominant dialogue in health-care settings, in which therapy often falls. Within this dialogue we see mixed opinions and arguments regarding how applicable the agenda is for the practice of therapy and mental health practice (Ramey and Grubb, 2009). Some of these issues raise questions such as: what should constitute evidence? Does empirical support translate into the best form of therapy for each individual? and are certain models of therapy better theoretically positioned to establish an evidence base?

These are big questions, and unfortunately do not come with a straightforward answer. It is important to acknowledge the EBP debate, but it is not our intention to quote the evidence base for each therapeutic model. Instead, we have chosen to designate the final chapter to showing how, as therapists, we can evidence the utility of our chosen therapeutic approach. Ultimately, we recommend thinking about what feels right for you as a therapist, and for the person accessing therapy.

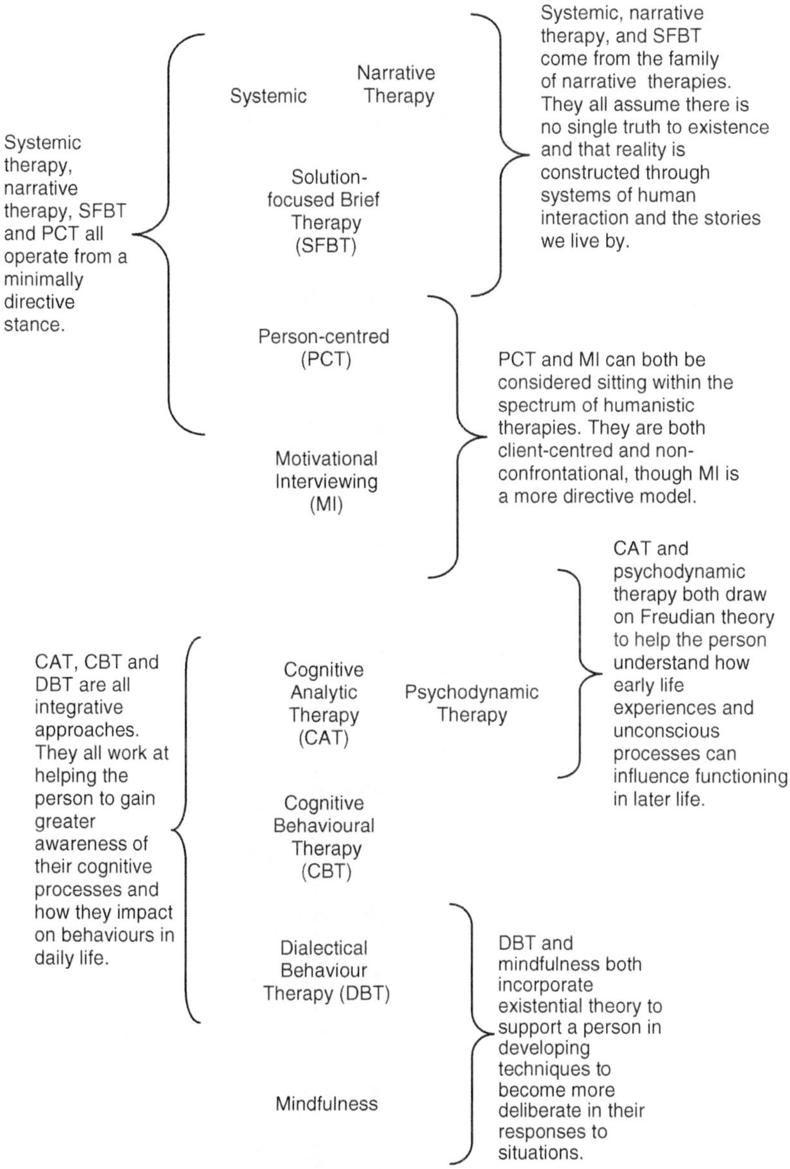


**Figure 1.1** The relationship between the ten therapeutic models discussed in this book

## THE THERAPEUTIC RELATIONSHIP

Regardless of model, the foundation of all therapy should be the therapeutic relationship. Clarkson (2003) describes 'relationship' as the first condition of being human, in that a relationship

> circumscribes two or more individuals and creates a bond in the space between them, which is more than the sum of parts.
>
> (Clarkson, 2003: 4)

When this unique bond sensitively meets the emotional needs of the person, it can be a powerful foundation for change to emerge. Lending from the work of John Bowlby (1988) we may consider the therapeutic relationship as the establishing of a secure base, from which the person can explore their inner world of thoughts, feelings and emotions. Many years of therapy-based research has shown that without establishing a good-quality therapeutic relationship, no model of therapy is likely to be received well, or applied successfully.

Some models of therapy (e.g. psychodynamic and person-centred therapy) have their own theoretical perspectives on the therapeutic relationship, which will be explored accordingly within their respective chapters. However, broadly speaking, there are some key features commonly considered by the psychotherapeutic community as being central to fostering a good therapeutic relationship (see Figure 1.2).

When considering the therapeutic relationship we must remember that being a good therapist does not mean being a perfect therapist. We are all human and as such we do, at times, behave in ways that place a strain on the therapeutic relationship. Perhaps something will be said that is upsetting for the person to hear, or we may misinterpret something the person has shared. Having these human moments is all part of the therapeutic process, and as Clarkson notes it is by

> working through these failures that the potential for healing and growth can emerge.
>
> (Clarkson, 2003: 136)

## DEVELOPING SKILLS FOR THERAPY

The road to becoming a competent therapist varies depending on professional background. However, whether training to be a counsellor, psychotherapist, clinical psychologist or other form of practitioner, we all have to develop skills in the particular model(s) of therapy that we wish to draw on. Understanding how we develop such skills can assist in our learning.

There are many models of learning, all of which are influenced by the issue at hand, our own belief systems, our abilities, the way in which we are taught, our goals, and of course the many factors tied up in the age-old nature–nurture

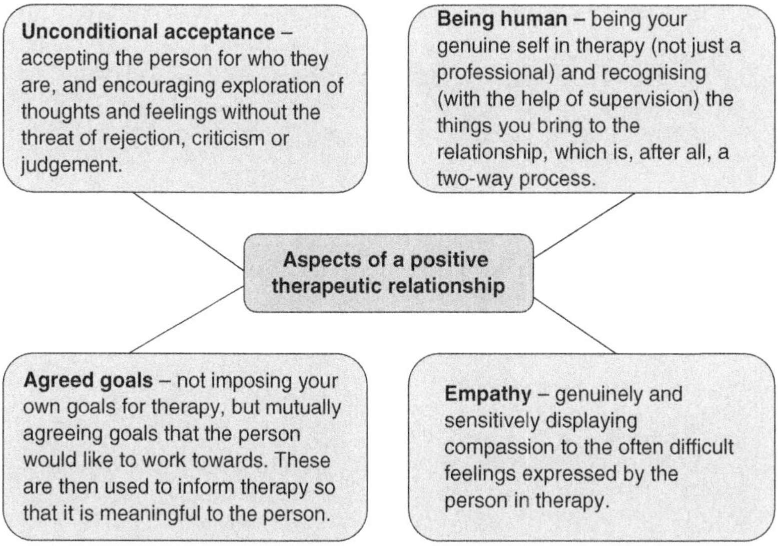


**Figure 1.2** The therapeutic relationship

debate. Learning about the theory and application of a therapeutic approach is as influenced by these factors as any other topic. Therapy is a powerful experience, both for the person accessing therapy and us as therapists. Therefore, when developing our therapeutic skills, it is important to think about all of these factors and try to have an understanding of where we are at in our own development.

One model for considering this issue is Maslow's theory of skill development (Maslow, 1987). This is a four-step model, describing the development of our awareness of our own ability levels. The idea is that we should move through different stages of competence in the topic at hand (in this case therapy), whilst also developing how conscious we are of our own skill-set. Figure 1.3 shows how it may look when applied to learning about a therapeutic approach.

This book will hopefully play a part in that development. In short, our intentions for the book are quite simple: to provide a clear and accessible 'pocket book guide' to applying the core models of therapy in practice. We hope that reading this book will increase your confidence and de-mystify the art of each therapeutic model, whilst helping you find the therapies that sit most comfortably with you and the people you help in therapy.

## REFERENCES

American Psychological Association (APA) (2005) *Policy Statement on Evidence-based Practice in Psychology*. Available at: www.apapracticecentral.org/ce/courses/ebpstatement.pdf (accessed 4 December 2010).

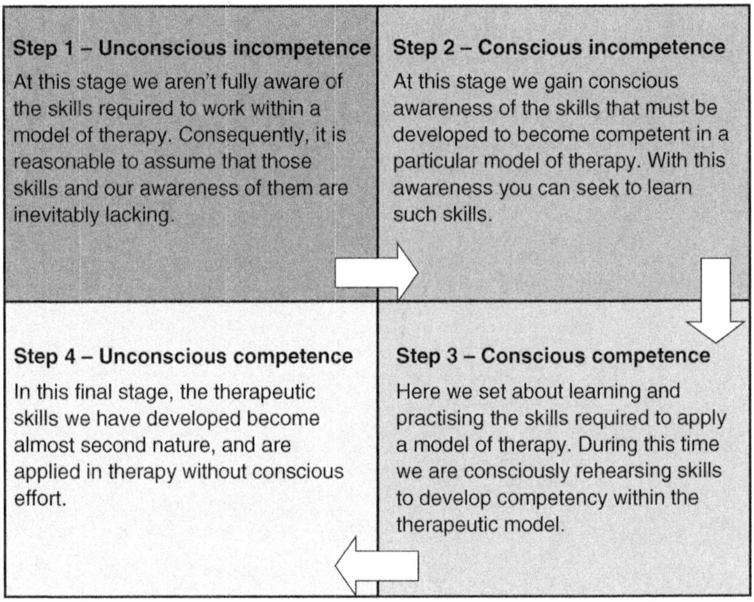


**Figure 1.3** Maslow's (1987) therapy of skill development applied to the therapeutic approach

American Psychological Association (APA) (2005) *Policy Statement on Evidence-based Practice in Psychology*. Available at: www.apapracticecentral.org/ce/courses/ebstatement.pdf (accessed 4 December 2010)

Bowlby, J. (1988) *A Secure Base*. London: Routledge.

Clarkson, P. (2003) *The Therapeutic Relationship*. London: Whurr.

House, R. (2003) *Therapy Beyond Modernity: Deconstructing and Transcending Profession-centred Therapy*. London: Karnac.

Johnstone, L. and Dallos, R. (2006) *Formulation in Psychology and Psychotherapy: Making Sense of People's Problems*. London: Routledge.

Maslow, A. H. (1987) *Motivation and Personality* (3rd edn). New York: Harper and Row.

Mithen, S. (1996) *The Prehistory of the Mind: A Search for the Origins of Art, Religion and Science*. London: Thames & Hudson.

Norcross, J. and Newman, C. F. (2003) 'Psychotherapy integration: Setting the context' in J. Norcross and J. C. Goldfried (eds), *Handbook of Psychotherapy Integration* (pp. 3–46). New York: Oxford University Press.

Palmer, S. (2000) *Introduction to Counselling and Psychotherapy: The Essential Guide*. London: Sage.

Ramey, H. L. and Grubb, S. (2009) 'Modernism, postmodernism and (evidence-based) practice', *Contemporary Family Therapy*, *31*, 75–86.

## NOTE

1. In the context of therapy and throughout this book, the term 'formulation' refers to the use of psychological theory to reach a provisional understanding of where the problem has originated from, and can be used to inform the process of therapy.

# 2 MOTIVATIONAL INTERVIEWING

Claire Robson

Motivational interviewing (MI) was initially developed for the treatment of people with alcohol problems. It has subsequently been used with a variety of problems, including drug abuse, gambling, eating disorders and lifestyle factors such as diet, exercise and smoking. MI can actually be applied to any problematic behaviour in which ambivalence for change is evident, which makes it applicable to a range of people accessing therapy. It directly addresses a significant problem common to many people and therapies – resistance to change. MI can be employed as a therapy in itself, in combination with other therapies or as an adjunct to other therapies. It can therefore serve as a valuable tool for all types of therapists, through fostering people's motivation to overcome their problems.

## THE MODEL

Motivational interviewing (MI) was developed by Miller (1983) and was later elaborated by Miller and Rollnick (1991). In the latest edition of their key text, Miller and Rollnick (2002: 25) defined MI as:

> A directive, client-centred counselling style for helping clients explore and resolve ambivalence about behaviour change.

Although like other therapies the goal is to facilitate change, MI differs in that it is more a way of 'being' with people rather than a distinct therapeutic approach. For the purposes of this chapter, it will be shown how MI can be used as a stand-alone treatment. However, hopefully it will still give you some insight into how you can use an 'MI style' when working with ambivalence and resistance in other forms of therapies.

The reasoning behind how MI appears to work is simple, but understanding the exact mechanisms remains a challenge. As human beings, we have an inherent desire to try to fix things and put things right. This desire can be stronger for some people, and is often what draws us into helping professions. It is therefore common and natural for therapists to feel frustrated when this does not happen, and to want to tell the person where they are going wrong. However, when a person with this 'righting reflex' meets a person who is ambivalent about change, the response is often resistance (e.g. disagreement, passivity or outright denial).

Therefore, at the heart of MI is the notion that 'the more a therapist tells a person that they desire change, the more the person will tell them why it can't happen'. In other words, progress in therapy is more likely to occur if motivation is not imposed on the person (e.g. by a confrontational interviewing style), but elicited intrinsically from the person. Indeed, the person needs to verbalise their own arguments for change.

Miller, who was a person-centred psychotherapist, advocated the use of empathic listening in order to minimise resistance and increase motivation for change. Although MI is considered to be a person-centred counselling style, it differs from traditional person-centred approaches in that it is directive rather than non-directive. Indeed, in MI there is a clear goal of exploring the person's ambivalence in a way that makes the person more likely to choose to change his/her behaviour. Systematic strategies are used in order to achieve this, and these will be explained in more detail in the Application section.

Before we move on to the 'how to' bit, it is important to highlight the three main concepts that have guided the development of MI:

1. **Readiness**: Motivation can be viewed as a state of readiness to change. The transtheoretical 'stages of change' model (Prochaska and Diclemente, 1984) describes a series of stages through which people pass as they change a behaviour. The model indicates that people have different needs depending on their stage of change. Although this model has also received some criticism over the years, it is still perhaps the most dominant and researched model of behaviour change.
2. **Ambivalence**: Often people have reasons why they want to change, but also why they don't. Holding opposing feelings about something is common, but when people become *stuck* in ambivalence it becomes a problem. The therapist's task in MI is to shift the balance of weights from the 'I don't want to' side to the 'I want to' side. People will then hear themselves (note – not their therapist) articulating their desire for change. These statements are likely to include indications that they feel ready, willing and able to change – the three critical components of motivation.
3. **Resistance**: In MI, the therapist always keeps in step with the person and their readiness to change in order to minimise resistance and facilitate the process of change. Resistance will be discussed in more detail throughout this chapter.

Prochaska and Diclemente's (1984) transtheoretical 'stages of change' model will be outlined in a bit more detail in the case example diagram at the end of this chapter.

## APPLICATION

### The spirit of MI

Miller and Rollnick contend that the underlying spirit of MI is vitally important in shaping the interview, perhaps even more so than the specific techniques that we'll look at later on. They believe that therapists can become too focused on matters of technique and lose sight of the spirit and style that are central to MI. So what is the spirit, I hear you say! The key components are outlined in Figure 2.1.

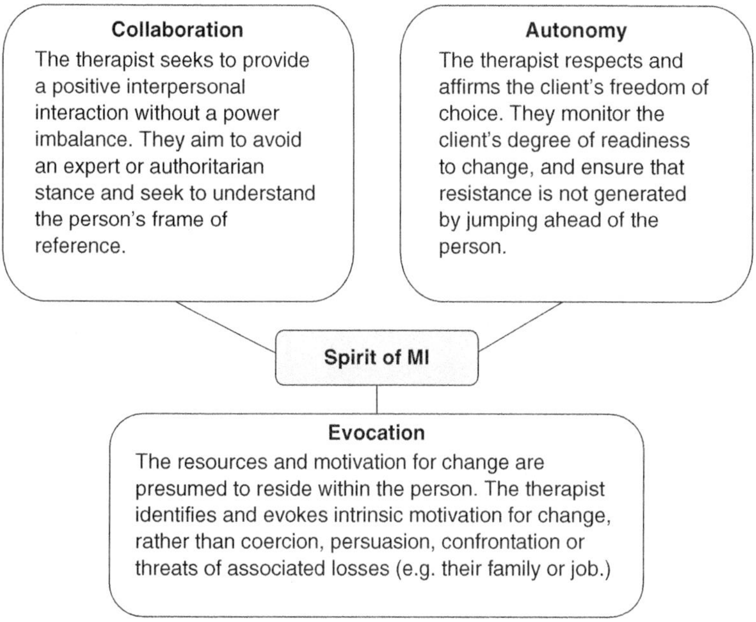


**Figure 2.1** The key components of the spirit of MI (Miller and Rollnick, 2002)

Miller and Rollnick argue that it is inappropriate to think of MI as a set of techniques that are applied to or used on people. It is an interpersonal style, shaped by an understanding of what triggers change. If it becomes a trick or manipulative technique, its essence has been lost.

### Principles of MI

Now that you've got the spirit, the next step is to consider the four main principles: expressing empathy, developing discrepancy, rolling with resistance and supporting self-efficacy.

> *Building Motivational Interviewing Skills* by Rosengren (2009) has some great ideas and examples of how you can practice interacting with people (including friends and family!) in an MI style.

1. **Expressing empathy**: An empathic, person-centred counselling style is seen as fundamental to MI. Reflective listening is used in order to understand the person's feelings and views, without judging or blaming (reflective listening will be explained more later). The attitude underlying the principle of empathy is one of acceptance, believing that ambivalence is a normal part of human experience and change.

2. **Developing discrepancy**: It is here where MI departs from more traditional person-centred approaches. MI helps people to move past ambivalence in the direction of helpful behaviour change. It is worth noting that the terms 'helpful' or 'positive' behaviour change in MI may open up an ethical dilemma for therapists, given that the person and their therapist may differ in their perceptions, goals and desire for change.

> If you're interested to hear more about the ethics of MI, have a read of Miller's (1994) paper dedicated to ethical issues within MI.

   Change is likely to arise when the person recognises that their target behaviour is inconsistent with the things they value as important to them. Miller predicts that unless there are things more important to the person than continuing the target behaviour, then motivational interviewing will not be effective. Indeed, 'motivation for change occurs when people perceive a discrepancy between where they are and where they want to be' (Miller et al. 1992: 8).

   It is important to explore the person's goals, values and aspirations for the future, and to highlight any discrepancies between these and the problem behaviour. Change is believed to be more likely to occur when this conflict is present. The result is generally that the person (not therapist) then presents the arguments for change.

3. **Rolling with resistance**: What we really don't do in MI is argue for change when the person is against it. Not only is the person unlikely to be persuaded, but it may actually make them want to do the opposite. There should not be a battle, and remember that it is not about winning or losing.

   In MI, resistance is not directly opposed, but rather acknowledged and explored, and is seen as a signal for the therapist to respond differently. The person is invited to consider new perspectives and information, but this is never imposed on them. Furthermore, therapists do not provide all the answers and solutions; instead, problems or questions are turned back to the person.

4. **Supporting self-efficacy**: Helping people to develop the belief 'I can do this' has long been recognised as a major element in motivation for change, making change more likely to happen. There is little point in just increasing a person's perception that they have a problem if the person perceives no hope for change, as no effort will be made. One of the goals of MI is therefore to enhance the person's confidence in their ability to succeed in change.

Holding both the spirit and principles of MI in mind, we will now explore the two main phases of how to apply MI in practice. Miller and Rollnick (2002) suggest there are two stages to MI work. Phase 1 aims to build intrinsic motivation to change (this is perhaps the most lengthy and arduous part). Once motivation reaches a certain point, it becomes important to move on to strategies for change (Phase 2). Phase 2 involves strengthening commitment to change and developing a plan of how to achieve change.

## PHASE 1 of MI – developing motivation to change

The amount of time spent on Phase 1 work depends on where the person is at when they start therapy. Some people may begin therapy with various reasons for change, whereas others may hardly be thinking about change.

To help understand how motivated the person is to change, it is useful to consider the person's confidence that change will happen, and also how important change is to them. Importance and confidence are both components of motivation to change and therefore are useful to assess. They can either be discussed informally with the person or by using rulers (see Worksheet 2.1 for rulers you can use in sessions).

Using the rulers, people are asked to rate importance and confidence on a scale of 0–10. The information gained can help you to decide what to prioritise in therapy. If both need to be addressed, the order depends on the person. Some people may need to address confidence first, such as those who have tried stopping their behaviour several times previously. Others may need to address importance first; however, for many both are addressed interchangeably.

### Techniques

There are four specific methods that are important to use right from the start and throughout MI. They are derived largely from person-centred counselling and can be easily remembered by the acronym OARS (**o**pen questions, **a**ffirmations, **r**eflections and **s**ummaries).

1. **Open questions** are questions that do not invite brief answers such as 'yes', 'no' or 'three years ago'. They are used in order to encourage the person to do most of the talking (very important in MI) and create a forward momentum that can be used to help the person explore change.

For example, you may want to begin the session with 'What brought you here today?' Perhaps later on you may want to say 'Could you tell me a little more about how your avoidance of going out is affecting your … ?'

2. **Affirmations** are a fantastic way of building rapport and reinforcing open exploration, providing that they come across as genuine and sincere. Affirmations may be in the form of compliments or statements of appreciation and understanding, for example 'That's a really good point' or 'You're the kind of person who cares a lot for other people'. Many people may have had very little experience of hearing these kinds of statements, so they can be particularly powerful.
3. **Reflections** or reflective listening is key component of MI, and is also perhaps the most challenging skill to learn. Reflective listening is a method of active listening, in which the therapist seeks to understand what the person means and then offers the idea back to the person in the form of a statement to check understanding. Basic reflections involve repeating, rephrasing or paraphrasing what the person has said, so that the person elaborates more. It is extremely important when making reflective statements to say them in flat tone of voice rather than question form. Note the difference between 'You're angry with your wife?' and 'You're angry with your wife.' The voice tone goes up at the end of a question but down at the end of a statement. Reflective listening statements therefore convey understanding rather than appearing challenging.

   Unlike in traditional Rogerian approaches, reflective listening in MI is used to actively guide the person towards certain topics. Not surprisingly, the therapist will give much more attention to statements that the person makes about wanting to change their behaviour. The following reflective statement illustrates this.

> Traditionally, reflective listening was used to facilitate discussion rather than guide the direction of discussion. For more information about the traditional use of reflective listening, see the work of Carl Rogers (e.g. Rogers, 1951).

**Example:** 'There are a few aspects of your drug use that you enjoy, but you have become increasingly concerned about its impact on your paranoid thoughts and memory.'

Reflections of affect are also particularly potent in motivating a person, particularly when the affect is not explicitly stated by the person. For example, if a person says 'My wife is going to leave me if I don't sort out my depression', a reflection of affect may be 'It sounds as though that bothers you a lot'.

Reflections are considered so crucial to MI that Miller and Rollnick advise a ratio of at least three reflections to one open question. So why more reflections than questions, given that therapists can never be sure whether their understanding is correct? Well, its simple: reflections are less likely to create resistance. Questions require responses and can stop momentum, whereas reflections facilitate forward momentum and keep it flowing in order to create change. In MI, specific types of reflections are used to respond to resistance when it occurs. These will be explained a little more later on, along with other techniques to minimise resistance.

4. **Summaries** are a type of reflective listening, where the therapist reflects back a summary of what the person has discussed. Summaries have multiple purposes, including showing the person that you're listening carefully, bringing attention to salient parts of the discussion, reinforcing what has been said and shifting the focus from one topic to another. Summaries can also link together what the person has just said with material from an earlier part of the session, or different session altogether. This can be particularly helpful in clarifying a person's ambivalence; for example, through allowing the person to vacillate back and forth between considering the pros and cons of change.

**Example:** Steve, 34, was a manager in a large consultancy company and was referred to the Community Alcohol Team by his GP, after he admitted a significant increase in his drinking over the past year due to stress at work. About half way through the first session, the therapist decided to use a summary to bring together some salient aspects of their discussion so far:

'I wonder if I could take a minute to check that I'm understanding things correctly. You've been under a huge amount of stress at work recently and you've found yourself out drinking for several hours every night and weekends, which you feel relaxes you and helps you to stop thinking about work. But you're concerned about how your drinking may now be affecting your relationship with your wife, who you care about a lot. You're also worried that you're not there for your children as much as you'd like to be. It sounds like it's a very difficult time in your life and you're thinking really hard about the best way to move forward.'

In using OARS to work through Phase 1, you may find it useful to use what is known as a 'decisional balance sheet' (see Worksheet 2.2 – 'Weighing up change') to facilitate exploration of ambivalence. This consists of a set of pros and cons for each of the options available to the person. Miller and Rollnick (2002) highlight the importance of not oversimplifying ambivalence by assuming that each advantage and disadvantage will have equal value, for example 'I know it's bad for my health, but I really enjoy it'. Elements in the sheets may also be related, for example a change in one can cause a change in another. Ambivalence can be a very complex and confusing experience.

However, in MI, OARS are not only used to help the person explore ambivalence, but also to direct the person towards change (see Worksheet 2.3 for example). OARS have the additional purpose of resolving ambivalence, by eliciting what is known as 'change talk' or 'self-motivational statements' from the person. Different types of change talk to look out for in people include:

- *Problem recognition* – 'I never really thought about how much worse my anorexia has got.'
- *Expression of concern about perceived problems* – 'I'm scared about what this could do to me.'
- *Intention to change* – 'I'm sick of feeling like this – I want to stop.'
- *Expressions of optimism about change* – 'I can do this.'

These statements can be difficult to hear, but whenever you do, *reflect, reflect, reflect.* Remember, the more people hear themselves talk about change, the more they'll hear the benefits (see Worksheet 2.4 for some more examples of change talk).

## Responding to resistance

Dealing with resistance uses some of the above techniques, but given how central resistance is to MI work (and the potential consequences of not responding to resistance appropriately) it warrants a section of its own. Table 2.1 therefore outlines some strategies for handling resistance from people, all of which follow the simple rule of responding to resistance with non-resistance.

## Confidence

Much of what we've discussed so far has focused on increasing a person's perceived importance of change, that is, whether they want to change. But remember the other key component in motivation is confidence, that is whether they feel able to change. Here are a few methods which can be helpful in eliciting and strengthening confidence talk. These are not necessarily MI-specific techniques (as with many of the techniques if applied without the spirit), but are useful within MI.

Open questions can be useful in eliciting confidence talk, such as: 'How might you begin to change – what would be a good place to start?' or 'What gives you a bit of confidence that you can change?' Alternatively, you could use the confidence ruler to rate how confident the person is from 0-10, then

| Strategy | Examples |
| --- | --- |
| **Simple reflection**<br>A simple reflective listening statement is one which repeats or rephrases what the person has just said | *James*: What's the point of talking about this? I can't stop – all my friends gamble.<br>*Therapist*: You feel like stopping gambling would be very difficult because you spend a lot of time with friends who gamble. |
| **Amplified reflection**<br>Another method is to reflect back what the person has said in an amplified or exaggerated form – without any hint of sarcasm. This often results in the person disagreeing with what you have said, eliciting the other side of their ambivalence. | *Lizzie*: I don't think anything will help now – it's probably too late.<br>Therapist: Maybe you're at the point of accepting that your relationship with your son is beyond repair. |
| **Double-sided reflection**<br>These are used to capture both sides of the person's ambivalence – the therapist presents both the resistant statement being made and contradictory material that the person has offered previously. | *Ella*: I know I use coke more than I should, but I don't use it all the time – I'm not addicted!<br>*Therapist*: I can see how this feels confusing for you. You've told me how you're concerned about how your coke use affects you, and also it seems like you're not using coke as much as some people. |
| **Shifting focus**<br>Another good way of dealing with resistance is to shift the focus of the discussion to another topic. | *Bobby*: I don't even want to be here – what can you tell me that I don't already know?<br>*Therapist*: I'm not here to give you advice, but what I can do is help you think more about your depression and what may be keeping it going. You were saying earlier that … |

*(Continued)*

**Table 2.1** Examples of reflective methods

*(Continued)*

| Strategy | Examples |
|---|---|
| **Agreement with a twist**<br>This is where the therapist agrees with most of the statement, but adds a slight twist or change of direction. | *Mike:* No-one can tell me what to do – you don't know what it's like having to live in my house.<br>*Therapist:* You're right, I don't know what it's like at all – only you know. You're in the best position to know which ideas are likely to work and which aren't. It's important that you decide what is best for you and your family. |
| **Reframing**<br>Another approach is to reframe what the person has said. This allows information to be viewed in a new light or reorganised form, which is likely to be more helpful and facilitate change. | *Peter:* He's always sticking his nose in and telling me I need to eat more, it really makes me angry.<br>*Therapist:* It sounds as if he really cares about you, to keep on trying to discuss this with you despite knowing that you'll get angry with him. |
| **Emphasising personal choice and control**<br>When a person perceives that their freedom of choice is threatened, they may be more likely to react by asserting their liberty and going against advice. We need to tell the person that it is *they* who determine what choice they make. | *Sam:* Why are you giving me this leaflet – are you trying to scare me into quitting?<br>*Therapist:* This is just information. What you do with it is entirely your choice. No-one can make you quit, you're a free person and it's your decision. |
| **Therapeutic paradox**<br>This strategy is often used with people who appear to oppose all suggestions made. The strategy is used with caution, as the idea is to recommend that the person continues or even increases their target behaviour (in a calm and matter-of-fact manner). This technique fits with the very nature of ambivalence – that when the therapist raises one side of ambivalence, the person is inclined to raise the other. | *Toni:* I know I shouldn't smoke as many cigs as I do, but I don't think it's that much of a problem.<br>*Therapist:* Perhaps it's not worth you stopping smoking, even though it causes you some problems – it's best to carry on as you are. |

**Table 2.1** Examples of reflective methods

ask follow-up questions such as these to elicit confidence talk, for example, 'Why are you at _____ and not ______?' and 'What would need to happen for you to go from _____ to ____ [a higher number on the scale]?'

Another method is to review the person's past successes and positive changes that they have made at previous points in their life. It's useful to elicit personal skills and strengths that can be generalised to their present situation. These strengths can then be explored and elaborated using reflective listening. Reflective listening remains a key technique here, so we use reflections to respond to confidence talk just as we would to change talk. Reframing can also be useful when people have tried to overcome problems several times but feel they have 'failed'. For example, failures can be reframed as 'tries' in order to support rather than block further attempts to change. Ideas for how to carry out change can be generated with the person, and should mainly come from the person.

## PHASE 2 of MI – strengthening commitment to change

Once intrinsic motivation to change is generated, which can take varying amounts of time depending on the individual, the next step is to strengthen commitment to change. So the million dollar question is: How do we know when a person is ready to change? A few indicators of a person's readiness for change are shown in Figure 2.2.

Not all of the indicators need to happen in each person, but they are good indicators that it might be time to shift the direction of therapy to a new goal of strengthening commitment to change. This can be a very exciting

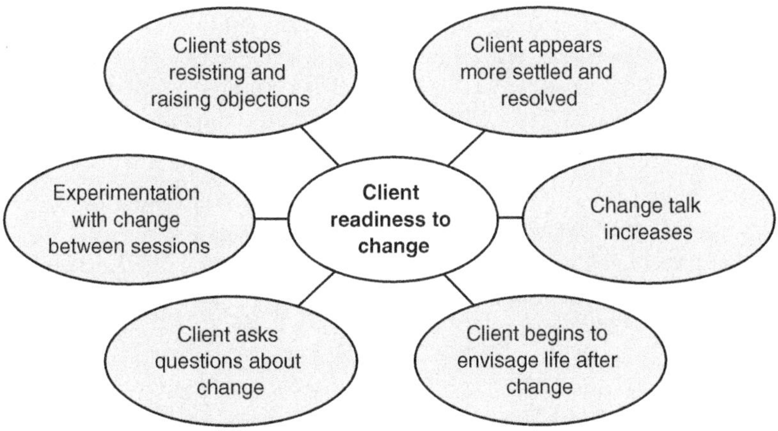


**Figure 2.2** Recognising a client's readiness to change

time. The next steps towards strengthening commitment include recapitulation, key questions, information and advice and negotiating a plan. Here is an outline of each step:

1. **Recapitulation** is basically a summary of what has been discussed so far, to draw together as many reasons for change as possible whilst acknowledging the other side of the person's ambivalence. It is used to ease the transition to the commitment phase and leads directly to some key questions.
2. **Key questions** are used to help people think about what they want and plan to do next. They are, of course, open questions such as 'Where do you think you can go from here?' and 'What are your options?' Once again, answers to these questions are responded to with reflective listening statements. This will facilitate further exploration and help the person to clarify their thoughts and plans.
3. **Information and advice** within MI, surprisingly, can be given to people, although only in two situations: i) when the person requests it, or ii) when the therapist obtains the person's permission to give it. This ensures that the spirit of MI (collaboration, evocation and autonomy) is maintained. For example, if a person asks for advice, the therapist could say something along the lines of 'I can tell you about some things that other people have found helpful, but I don't know if they'll be right for you.' If the therapist feels that there is important information that they need to give to a person and they have already elicited the person's own ideas and knowledge, they can ask permission to give advice (note – therapists can only give advice if these two prior conditions are met).

   **Example:** Natasha, 28, had an appointment with her practice nurse. Natasha told the nurse that she was thinking about giving up smoking because of concerns about the health risks of smoking around her young daughter. However, she was worried that if she did give up smoking then she would put on weight. The nurse thought this could be an important opportunity to give Natasha some information about smoking cessation and weight gain:

   'I wonder if it would be useful for me to give you some information which might help with your concerns about gaining weight after stopping smoking? ... How much weight do you think the average person gains in their first year of quitting? ... Would you be interested to know the results of some research about this?'

4. **Negotiating a plan** is the next step as hopefully by now a plan for change will be developing. Remember that motivation occurs when people develop a discrepancy between their current situation and where they want to be. Goal setting is therefore essential to help the person

to consider how they would like things to be different, what they want to change and what areas should be prioritised. A variety of change options are then generated and evaluated, before reaching an explicit change plan.
The final step is to elicit commitment from the person to the change plan, often simply by asking 'Is this what you want to do?' If the answer is 'Yes', then our work is done. If the person is unsure, then the change plan may need to be amended or some more Phase 1 work on resolving ambivalence may be necessary.

> Miller and Rollnick's website: www.motivationalinterview.org contains additional resources (including change plans) that can be used in sessions, along with further very accessible information about the approach in general.

Once commitment is attained, many people are able to carry out the changes by themselves. It can be particularly helpful for the person to share their change plan with family or friends to elicit support. Moreover, the more the person verbalises the plan to others, the more commitment is strengthened. If necessary and appropriate, other therapies (such as the many within this book) could be used to help people carry through with change.

So that's MI in a nutshell. Hopefully this will have whetted your appetite to use MI within your practice and/or to do some further reading and training. Enjoy!

## CASE STUDY

Sarah, a 23-year-old female, was referred by her general practitioner (GP) for help with managing her alcohol use. The referral stated that she had presented to the GP with pains around her abdomen, which he felt was due to problematic levels of drinking. The GP said that Sarah had agreed to attend a consultation to discuss her drinking further.

Sarah attended an initial assessment appointment, brought by her mother who stayed in the waiting room. Sarah initially reported feeling unsure why the GP had suggested that she attend the clinic, as she described her drinking as 'no worse than most people my age'. She acknowledged that on occasions she drank more than she intended and would often have stomach cramps after heavy drinking

*(Continued)*

*(Continued)*

sessions, but felt that other people had more of a problem with it than she did. She appeared reluctant to be at the clinic, and angrily stated that 'It's my business, other people always have to stick their noses in'.

It was clear that Sarah had come into the session armed with an argument against change, and it would have been very easy for the therapist to challenge her views and end up in an argumentative 'confrontation/denial' trap. However, given Sarah's high level of resistance at the start, it was important for the therapist to 'roll' with it and spend most of the first session using reflective listening statements to acknowledge and explore her feelings and views. This enabled Sarah to become visibly more relaxed, and she even expressed feeling surprised that she was not being 'given a lecture' as she had expected. The therapist explained that this was not his role and that it was entirely up to her what she decided to do.

A turning point in the session occurred when an amplified reflection was used by the therapist to reflect how it seemed to Sarah that other people had no reason for concern about her drinking. Sarah was then able to say how her drinking sometimes led to arguments with her parents, who were concerned about her health. She said that they would also often shout at her for staying out late and getting in trouble. Further exploration of the above using reflective listening and open questions led her to describe how she could get 'loud and bolshie' when she drank and how she had fallen out with friends as a result. She also explained how there had been a few times where she had got into fights with people and how the police had been called on one of these occasions.

Sarah agreed to come back to the clinic the following week. Over the next few sessions both sides of Sarah's ambivalence were explored using OARS. Sarah described working in a bar in town and how her drinking had escalated because it was common for staff to drink during shifts. They would also often stay for drinks after work or go out to other local bars. A double-sided reflection enabled her to consider how on the one hand she felt her drinking was 'social' and enabled her to 'have a laugh' at work, but on the other hand she felt that her drinking had begun to have a damaging impact on her relationships with her friends and parents. She also described how the bar manager had told her off recently for 'getting mouthy' and being rude to a customer. As a result, she had been told that if she did this again she may lose her job. She expressed concern that she had no savings as she was spending most of the money she earned on alcohol, so would have no money if she lost her job.

Change talk was elicited and reflected, with the aim of building intrinsic motivation for change. At session five, the therapist considered whether to continue with Phase 1 methods or to go onto Phase 2 and begin work on strengthening commitment to change and discussing strategies. The therapist looked for indicators of readiness. Sarah was considerably less resistant than in session one, and had begun to consider what life would be like if she did not drink as much. There had even been a couple of nights where she had gone out after work but only had one drink, and she expressed feeling glad to have a bit of spare cash at the end of the week. However, she expressed concern that she would really struggle to say no to offers of drinks at work, when she didn't have to pay for drinks. Sarah felt drinking at work was the biggest trigger to her alcohol use. Given this, and that most of the alcohol she drank was at work, time was spent first focusing on her confidence to change this aspect of her drinking.

Once confidence talk began to emerge, the therapist then decided to test Sarah's readiness by asking Sarah where she wanted to go from here (a 'key question' regarding change). Sarah said that she wanted to do something about her drinking, but stated a preference to cut down rather than stop altogether. The therapist helped her to think about both of these methods of change, without giving advice. However, Sarah then asked the therapist's opinion on what she should do. The therapist was then able to suggest to Sarah that, given her stomach cramps, it may be best for her to have at least a period of abstinence to help her body recover. However, it was emphasised to Sarah that the ultimate decision was hers. Sarah and the therapist were then able to write out a change plan, which included a six-month break from drinking (see Figure 2.3). A range of options to help her carry out the plan were explored. Sarah decided to access help from her parents but felt that she would not need any further help from services. Three and six-month follow-up appointments were arranged, and at both points she had not drunk any alcohol. Her stomach pains ceased and after six months she was applying for different jobs so that she would no longer be working in a pub environment. She still intended to start drinking socially again once she had moved jobs, but wanted to minimise triggers for relapse first.

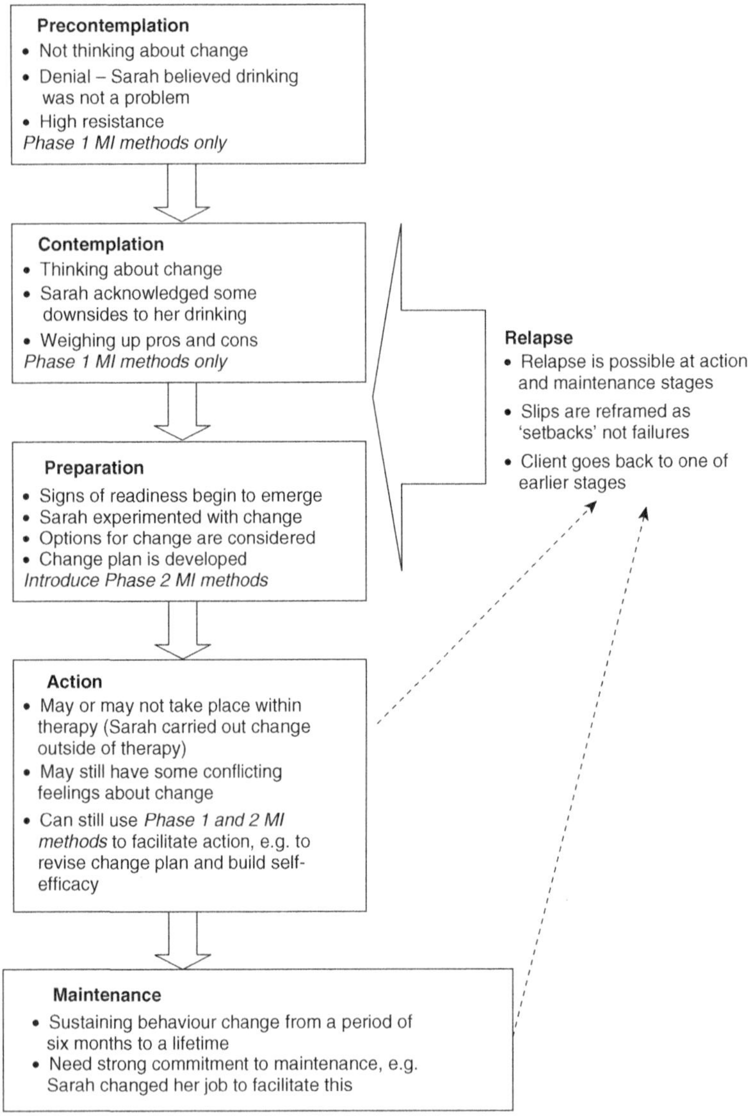


**Figure 2.3** Diagrammatic formulations are not used in Motivational Interviewing, however the following is based on the 'stages of change' model (Prochaska and Diclimente, 1984) with a consideration of some of the characteristics of each stage in Sarah's case.

## GLOSSARY

| | |
|---|---|
| Affirmations | Compliments or statements of appreciation and understanding. |
| Ambivalence | Feeling two ways about something – 'I want to, but I don't want to'. |
| Change plan | This refers to an explicit plan detailing how change can be carried out, and is established either verbally or in a written format. |
| Change talk | Statements about change made by a person, including expressions of problem recognition, concerns about their problems, intention to change and optimism about change. |
| Client-centred counselling | A counselling approach developed by Carl Rogers, in which the person determines the general direction of sessions rather than the therapist. Empathy, warmth and genuineness are viewed as critical in facilitating a safe and supportive atmosphere in which natural change can occur. |
| Confrontational interviewing style | The opposite of motivational interviewing – therapists push people towards making changes for which they are not ready, thus creating high levels of resistance. |
| Developing discrepancy | This refers to how motivation arises by developing a discrepancy between where a person is now and where they want to be. |
| Expressing empathy | Empathy refers to the process of seeking to understand and accept the person's feelings and views. Empathy is expressed using OARS (Open questions, Affirmations, Reflections and Summaries). |
| Key questions | These are questions often asked in Phase 2 of motivational interviewing to help people think about what they want and plan to do next. |
| Motivation (components of) | Three critical components of motivation include readiness, willingness and ability (confidence) to change. |
| Open questions | Questions that do not invite brief answers such as 'yes', 'no' or 'next year'. |
| OARS | Acronym used to remember four techniques used within MI – Open questions, Affirmations, Reflections and Summaries. |

| | |
|---|---|
| Reflective listening | This is a method of active listening, in which the therapist seeks to understand the person's feelings and views and then offers the idea back to the person *in the form of a statement* to check understanding. |
| Recapitulation | A summary of what has been discussed so far, which often draws together as many reasons for change as possible whilst acknowledging the other side of the person's ambivalence. |
| Rolling with resistance | This refers to how resistance is responded to with non-resistance rather than opposition; the therapist is always trying to stay alongside the person. |
| Self-motivational statements | See 'Change talk'. |
| Summaries | A type of reflective listening, where the therapist reflects back a summary of what the person has discussed. |
| Supporting self-efficacy | The therapist aims to enhance the person's confidence in their ability to succeed in change, to make change more likely to happen. |
| The righting reflex | This refers to our natural desire to 'put things right', e.g. through giving advice, teaching or arguing for change. If ambivalence is met in this way, resistance is often created. |

## REFERENCES


Miller, W. R. (1983) 'Motivational Interviewing with problem drinkers', *Behavioural Psychotherapy, 11*, 147-172.

Miller, W. R. (1994) 'Motivational Interviewing: III. On the ethics of motivational intervention', *Behavioural and Cognitive Psychotherapy, 22*, 111-123.

Miller, W. R. and Rollnick, S. R. (1991) *Motivational Interviewing: Preparing People to Change Addictive Behaviour.* New York: Guilford Press.

Miller, W. R. and Rollnick, S. R. (2002) *Motivational Interviewing: Preparing People for Change* (2nd edn). New York: Guilford Press.

Miller, W. R., Zweben, A., Diclemente, C. C. and Rychtarik, R. (1992) *Motivational Enhancement Therapy Manual: A Clinical Research Guide for Therapists Treating Individuals with Alcohol Abuse and Dependence* (Project MATCH Monograph Series, Vol. 2). Rockville, MD: National Institute on Alcohol Abuse and Alcoholism.

Motivational Interviewing website: *Motivational Interviewing – Resources for Clinicians, Researchers and Trainers, www.motivationalinterview.org/.*

Prochaska, J. O. and Diclemente, C. C. (1984) *The Transtheoretical Approach: Crossing the Traditional Boundaries of Therapy.* Malabar, FL: Krieger.

Rogers, C. R. (1951) *Client-centred Therapy: Its Current Practice, Implications and Theory.* London: Constable.

Rosengren, D. B. (2009) *Building Motivational Interviewing Skills: A Practitioner Workbook.* New York: Guilford Press.

# Worksheet 2.1

## Importance and confidence rulers

How important is it for you to change your ____________[target behaviour]?

0 1 2 3 4 5 6 7 8 9 10

| Not important at all | Extremely important |
|---|---|

How confident are you in change your ____________[target behaviour]?

0 1 2 3 4 5 6 7 8 9 10

| Not important at all | Extremely important |
|---|---|

Some useful additional questions:

- Why did you give yourself a score of ____ and not ____[lower]?
- What would need to happen for your score to move up from a ____ to a ____ [higher]
- How might your life be different if you moved from a ____ to a ____ [higher]?
- What could you do to increase the importance/confidence about changing your __________ [target behaviour]?

## Worksheet 2.2

## Weighing up change

What may be also referred to as 'decisional balance sheets' are essentially a means of helping the person to weigh up the pros and cons of change. This can then be used as motivation to continue with change at times of difficulty. Use this worksheet to weigh up whether to keep the target behaviour or engage in change.

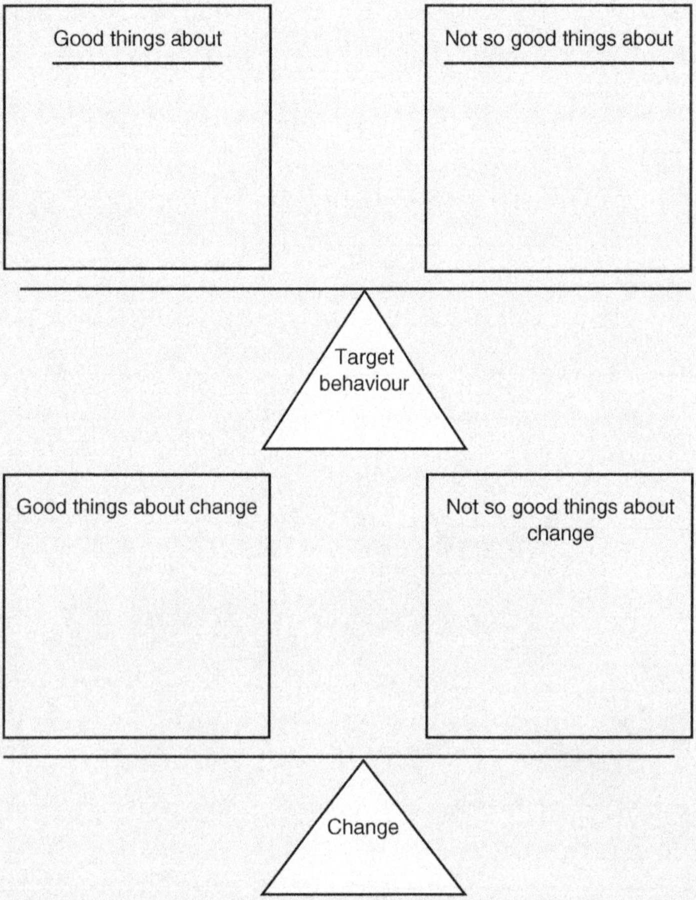

# Worksheet 2.3

## (OARS) Open questions, Affirmations, Reflections and Summaries)

| | What are they? | Examples |
|---|---|---|
| Open questions | Questions that do not invite brief answers such as 'yes', 'no'. They are used to encourage the person to do most of the talking and create a forward momentum that can be used to help the person explore change. | • 'How has the problem impacted on your life?'<br>• 'In what ways would you like the problem to change?'<br>• 'What would be different if the problem was not around anymore?' |
| Affirmations | A way of building rapport and reinforcing open exploration, providing that they come across as genuine and sincere. Affirmations may be in the form of compliments or statements of appreciation and understanding. | • 'That's a really good point.'<br>• 'I can see that is really important to you.'<br>• 'It sounds like that was a really difficult experience. '<br>• 'You're the kind of person who cares a lot for other people.' |
| Reflective listening | A method of active listening whereby the therapist seeks to understand what the person means and then offers the idea back to the person (in a flat tone) in the form of a statement to check understanding. | • 'The depression has taken many things away from you and your family.'<br>• 'You feel as though avoiding stressful situations doesn't help, but it's hard to know what else to do.' |
| Summaries | A type of reflective listening, where the therapist reflects back a summary of what the person has discussed. | • 'I wonder if I could take a minute to check that I'm understanding things correctly ...'<br>• 'So it sounds like you are saying that ... does that capture what we have just discussed?' |

# Worksheet 2.4

## Change talk

Spotting 'change talk' in therapy can be an important indicator that the person has begun to resolve ambivalence towards change. Below are four common types of change talk with some examples of how they may be phrased by the person in therapy. Remember to reflect any change talk back to the person so they can hear the benefits of change.

**Change talk**

**Problem recognition**
Where the person recognises the problem and/or the effect it is having on their life.

- *I never really thought about how much worse [the problem] has gotten.*
- *[The problem]has taken over my life.*
- *[The problem]has stopped me from ...*

**Expression of concern about problems**
Concern for the effect the problem is having on self or others.

- *I'm worried [the problem] will cause me to ...*
- *I'm concerned about the effect [the problem] is having on my family and friends.*

**Intention to change**
Any comment that demonstrates intent to change the current problem.

- *I would like to start ...*
- *I just want to be able to ...*
- *I'm fed up of ... and just want to ...*
- *I'm sick of feeling like this – I want to stop.*

**Expressions of optimism about change**
Comments that show a sense of hope that change is possible.

- *I suppose it's possible that ...*
- *I might be able to ...*
- *I can do this.*

# 3 COGNITIVE BEHAVIOURAL THERAPY

Jane Toner

Cognitive behavioural therapy (CBT) is an active, directive, time-limited and structured therapeutic approach to mental health problems and distress. Therapy is based upon a collaborative and open relationship between the therapist and the person accessing therapy using explorative questions and specific techniques. Within this context 'cognitive' refers to our thoughts, images and interpretations that occur within and beyond our stream of consciousness. 'Behaviour' refers to our behaviour and actions.

## THE MODEL

The principle theoretical rationale underpinning cognitive behavioural therapy (CBT) was first discussed by Aaron Beck in the 1960s. CBT is built on the concept that the interaction of feelings and behaviour is dependent on how we interpret any given situation. No two people will interpret a situation in exactly the same way. Let us take the example of two people being given a skydive as a surprise gift. The first person may think 'Fantastic, how generous, I can't wait for it' – they would probably feel excited, happy and look forward to the event. The second person may think 'Oh no, how scary, why did they buy this for me?' – this person could experience feelings of apprehension, fear and maybe even annoyance, and may ultimately try to avoid the skydive. This different interpretation and reaction to the same event can be explained through considering their past experiences, cognitive make-up and their beliefs (about themselves, their world and others).

### The cognitive model

A number of specific cognitive processes are thought to make up the cognitive model. They are deeper-level core beliefs, conditional beliefs and lastly automatic beliefs or thoughts. Information processing in relation to maintaining and reinforcing these beliefs is also fundamental to the model and will be discussed.

> CBT has developed over the years in many therapeutic areas. If you want to read more about these developments, an overview is provided at the end of the chapter.

*Core beliefs* are placed at the deepest level of functioning (also known in some literature as 'schema'). These can be understood as a relatively stable set of beliefs, which are basic and extreme, developed early on in life, and are reinforced through experience. They are also known as 'unconditional' because they tend to be accepted as fact by the individual and are difficult to dispute. Core beliefs formed during traumatic events are thought to be the most difficult to change and adapt.

We all view situations differently, but each of us tends to be consistent in the way that we personally conceptualise events and situations, therefore core beliefs can be thought of as a consistent way of thinking in different environments. Many core beliefs are functional and useful, but some are negative and problematic and cause some of us difficulties at times. It is important to acknowledge that core beliefs are generally formed in response to our environments and our experiences of others. They have therefore served a contextual purpose at some point (maybe during early experiences or when under threat).

Core beliefs are thought to influence the type of information we seek, what we focus on, and what we accept more easily. As a result, they are readily and repeatedly reinforced. Because our core beliefs shape how we interpret situations and experiences, they affect our behaviour and mood. Some particular core beliefs can be inactive for a long time, but can become powerful again when specific memories are triggered. For example, during a period of stress or trauma in adult life, some beliefs or schema formed in childhood such as 'I am vulnerable' may be re-triggered or reinforced, and may begin to play a part in how the adult interprets their future experiences. This may also end up being generalised to other aspects of life.

Core beliefs can be described as a 'cognitive triad'. As shown in Figure 3.1, this represents three major cognitive patterns related to how people view themselves, the world and the future. For example, a depressed person may think:

- They are undesirable and worthless, 'I am …'
- Others are difficult and challenging, 'Others are …'
- Their difficulties will continue indefinitely, 'The future is …'

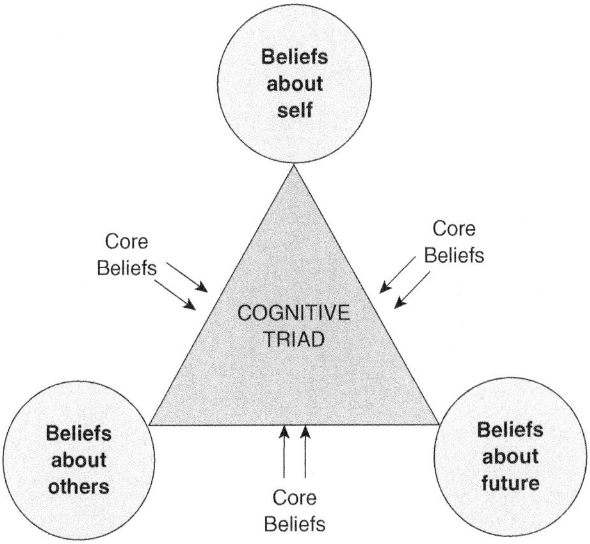


**Figure 3.1** The cognitive triad

*Conditional beliefs* (also known in the literature as 'rules for living') are the next level of beliefs and are thought to be more in our awareness. They are often linked with the basic schema. They involve assumptions or short-cuts about how we carry out our lives and our relationships and ways of functioning. They are intended to help us get our needs met and cope with life. They may exist in the form of assumptions, for example 'If I please her all the time, she'll like me.' They may also be in the form of a rule for living involving 'shoulds, musts and oughts', for example 'I must be liked by everyone', 'I should be able to manage this situation', 'I should be happy.'

*Automatic thoughts and beliefs* are those thoughts that occur more within our awareness, on a day-to-day basis. They can be described as occurring spontaneously/automatically, can occur within the therapy setting, and are often negative or problematic in content (they are often referred to as 'negative automatic thoughts' or NATs). Automatic thoughts, be they positive, neutral or negative, directly influence our behaviour, mood and physiology, which in turn act to reinforce the beliefs. Automatic thoughts can't be switched off consciously, and although they are often referred to as 'thoughts', they can be an image, verbal or pre-verbal (a sense or a 'feeling' about something). They represent how a person perceives things and are likely to reflect their underlying core beliefs.

Terminology such as 'thinking errors' and 'dysfunctional thinking' continue to be used in CBT literature. However, 'biases' may be a more helpful and less derogatory term. As therapists we need to be aware of the language we are using and how that language we use may be interpreted by the people we work with.

The final cognitive aspect to discuss is *information processing*. This involves interpreting or processing stimuli in a biased way, for example by actively noticing and selectively attending to negative feedback and ignoring or dismissing positive stimuli/information. This biased processing or interpretation of environmental stimuli acts to reinforce and maintain any problematic beliefs and behaviours that a person is engaging in. These 'biases' or extreme styles of processing affect the interpretation of events. This is likely to be in a way that is consistent with underlying beliefs, thereby reinforcing them. Broadly speaking, the interpretations of a person with low mood may be more extreme, negative, categorical, absolute and judgemental than someone else. CBT is aimed at helping a person to recognise these biases. Identifying why and how they have emerged should help to reduce biases and facilitate more rational, grounded interpretations of a situation.

In summary, a person's emotions and their behaviours are largely determined by the way in which they cognitively structure the world. They reflect the person's core beliefs of themselves, others, their past and future. Once activated, core beliefs lead to assumptions about self and other's worth and behaviours; they influence our day-to-day cognitions and ways of processing the stimuli in the environment (see Figure 3.2).

## APPLICATION

CBT is a structured therapeutic approach to working with individuals with mental health problems and distress. The techniques discussed below have been separated into the three key areas for practising CBT. These are: relationship development and the Socratic process; socialising and formulating; and cognitive and behavioural techniques. These three areas are all interlinked, so in CBT one cannot be practised without the other and high-quality CBT would involve them all.

### The therapeutic relationship and the Socratic process

CBT has been erroneously described as being predominantly technique-based, to the detriment of the therapeutic relationship, but this is far from the case. Aaron Beck stated that:

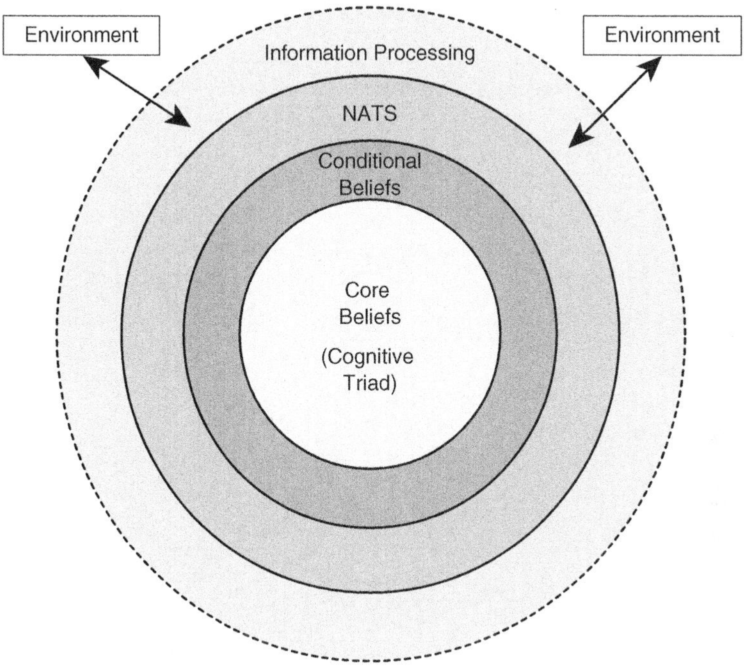


**Figure 3.2** Beliefs, thoughts and information processing

> The aspiring cognitive therapist must be first, a good psychotherapist, no matter how proficient he is in the technical application of cognitive strategies, he will be severely hampered if he is not adequately endowed with essential personal characteristics such as concern, genuineness and empathy.
>
> (Beck et al., 1979: 25)

He also emphasised the fact that CBT can only be practised in a 'collaborative' way, based on a partnership between the person accessing therapy and the therapist. There remains a debate about what specific aspects of the therapeutic relationship in CBT effect engagement and outcome (for a review, see Waddington, 2002), but CBT therapists need to be able to genuinely convey to people that they are trying to understand what they are feeling. The therapist needs to empathise with the meanings a person gives to events and try to view the world from their perspective. This involves going back to the basic elements of a therapeutic relationship, such as listening, conveying empathy, being honest and open.

The Socratic process is a form of dialogue that sets out to help a person discover and attend to new or overlooked material. The therapist's objective is to 'guide discovery', not to change the person's mind. This needs to be done in a positive, curious and supportive way. This should empower the person to find more helpful, balanced and functional ways of being. The following points from Christine Padesky (1993) provide a description of the four stages to the *guided discovery process*: ask information questions; listen; summarise; and use and synthesising or analytical questions.

1. **Ask information questions:** Questions should be relevant. The answer should be known to the person and be helpful. These questions should help concerns and problems become concrete and understandable.

   **Examples:**

   - When did these problems start?
   - How do you feel when this happens?
   - Which bit about this situation bothers you the most?
   - Why do you think this happens?

2. **Listen:** You must be listening to discover and understand the other person's experience. This will facilitate a natural surprise when you hear the unexpected. You also need to listen for particular words and how someone phrases something – they won't use textbook phrases. Listen out for emotional changes and for things that don't sound right or that don't seem congruent.
3. **Summarise:** This should be done regularly to check meaning and slow things down. It reinforces ideas being discussed and highlights things that have been discovered or concluded. It can also be a useful way to synthesise new information and look at things as a whole.

   **Example:** 'OK, so you've just told me that when you are out in public you become very aware of what is happening to you inside. You become hot, sweaty, feel sick, feel lightheaded, and you think that people can see that you are very red, embarrassed and shaking? Does that sound right?'

4. **Use synthesising or analytical questions:** You should ask these kinds of questions to apply what has been 'discovered' in relation to the initial concerns, beliefs and problems being discussed. These kinds of questions are very important, but difficult. As a result they are often neglected. The questions should promote objectivity and encourage someone to adopt a critical stance in relation to their patterns of thinking and behaving. This should facilitate new or alternative explanations and solutions.

**Example:** 'Based on what we have just discussed, are there any other ways that could explain what is happening?'

In Table 3.1, Christine Padesky (1993) describes four types of questions that are vital in this process and that are questions used throughout the conversations you have in each session.

Throughout the sessions you should be summarising what has been said, to show what you've heard and to check understanding. This can help to highlight key issues. Reflecting back what you have heard and what seems to be salient helps to focus attention on relevant things. This can also be a useful way of recognising and exploring patterns and connections. Validating what somebody has said or how they have expressed a feeling acknowledges their distress and their personal experience and can continue to build a relationship to enable therapeutic work.

| Question type | Summary | Examples |
|---|---|---|
| **Information gathering** | The person should always have the information within them to answer the questions you ask. These questions should enhance the therapeutic relationship, and be answerable with thought and attention. | Can you think back and tell me about a time when you haven't felt this way? What would be so bad if this belief were true? |
| **Attention drawing** | These should be relevant to the issue at hand, but be outside the current focus. They should trigger a retrieval of information. As the therapist you don't need to have the answers, but you do need to know where your questioning is heading. | I'm interested to know how these difficulties began? How frequently do you think these thoughts come and go on a daily basis? |
| **Switching between abstract and concrete** | Start with a question that defines the problem. Follow up with questions that foster new learning (these can generate experiments/ home tasks). | Can you describe a specific time when this feeling of anxiety was particularly strong? |
| **Re-evaluating** | Use new or previously overlooked information to re-evaluate a previous belief, or construct a new one. | You said that you don't go out anymore. But you do feel strong enough to visit this friend sometimes. What makes the difference? |

**Table 3.1** Questioning methods relevant to the guided discovery process (Padesky, 1993)

## Socialising and formulation

'Socialising' is a term used for the first session(s) of CBT where you are trying to promote and 'sell' the potential benefits of the model to the person. It involves gathering pertinent information and introducing the key aspects of the model. This may involve giving some information about CBT (psychoeducation), discussing each other's role in therapy and jointly developing an early formulation. Another aim of socialisation is to develop a joint understanding of the difficulties the person is experiencing. This can further increase motivation for therapy and improve their ability to cope with problems.

One way to introduce the CBT model is to ask the person to describe a problematic situation within the 'five systems' model (Greenberger and Padesky, 1995):

1. The environment.
2. Thoughts.
3. Feelings/mood.
4. Behaviour.
5. Physical aspects/physiology.

See also Figure 3.3 for a visual approach.

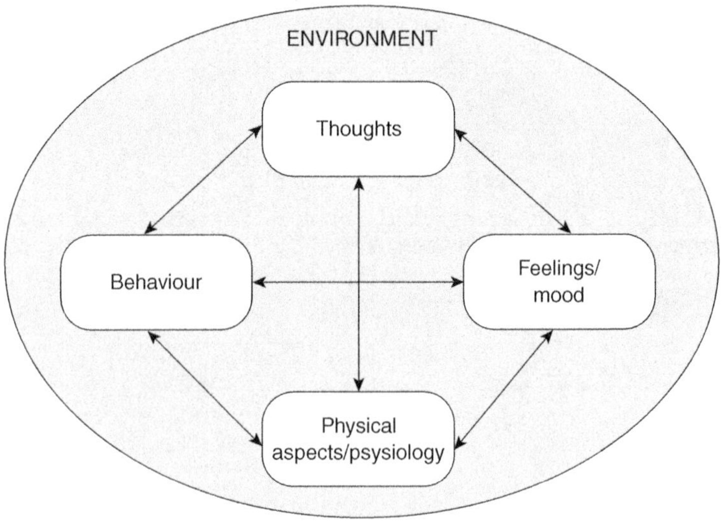


**Figure 3.3** The five systems model (Greenberger and Padesky, 1995)

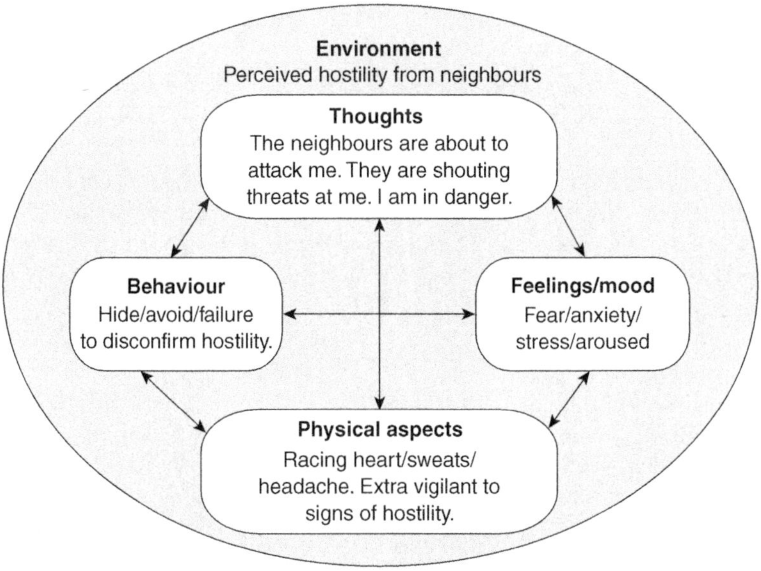


**Figure 3.4** Case example demonstrating the 5 systems model (Greenberger and Padesky, 1995)

During this process draw the person's attention to how each area is related, for example how the social/environmental aspects influence our mood and our behaviour, or how behaviour can influence mood.

You can explore together how thoughts and interpretations affect behaviour, motivation, physiology and mood. You can discuss how these effects would not be a problem if they happened in isolation or just faded away. Instead these thoughts tend to influence subsequent thoughts and emotions and therefore problems are maintained or can be exacerbated. This can be drawn out as a maintenance cycle to demonstrate the cyclical, reinforcing effect (or formulation – see Figure 3.4).

**Example:** Jimmy is a 38-year-old man who has been having paranoid thoughts since his early teens. Following a traumatic upbringing in which he was the victim of abuse from family members and neighbours, he began to view the world as a dangerous place and became fearful of expressing his feelings. He saw himself as a bad person and believed that if things went wrong they were his fault. He had also learned that to express his feelings often resulted in rejection.

Exploring and understanding how the different aspects of this formulation are related and linked can help us find ways to begin the process of change. You can also discuss how small changes in any one of the five areas can lead to changes in the other areas, giving a direction for intervention.

A formulation in CBT can be defined as a shared or joint understanding of the origins, the development and ongoing maintenance of a person's problem. It should guide the process of therapy, shaping assessment information into a theoretical format and guiding intervention. The process should be collaborative and descriptive. It should be based around the cognitive model, but use the person's own words, meanings and descriptions.

Formulations can be used to highlight relationships between different elements of the model, as well as considering how things have developed and changed over time. They are used to describe different patterns and traps, in order to make sense of them. The formulation provides a format to incorporate CBT theory into the session, and to structure the information being discussed. Finally, the formulation should provide a way forward through interventions that might be helpful, and ideas of where to intervene. It is important to keep things as simple as possible and not overwhelm the cognitive or emotional capacity of the person you are working with.

There are many different types of formulation used for different purposes and at various stages in the therapy sessions. Mini formulations can be used, often early on in therapy, to demonstrate or draw out the relationship between components of the basic cognitive model.

**Example:** Marie has a diagnosis of depression. One symptom of the depression is that she is less active. This reduced activity leads to increased levels of depression (see Figure 3.5).

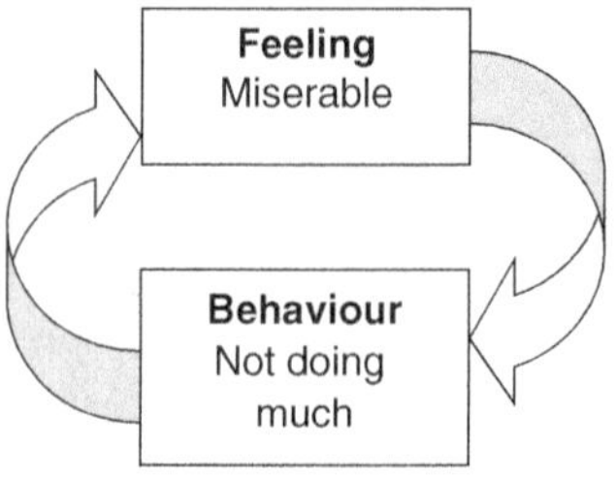


**Figure 3.5** The depressive cycles

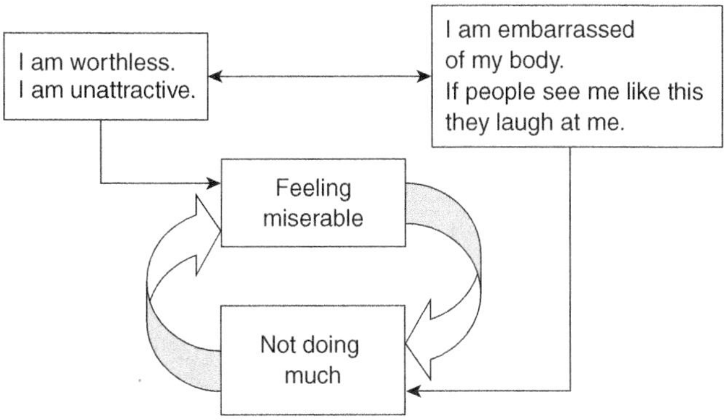


**Figure 3.6** A 'depression' mini formulation

Mini formulations can also be drawn out between day-to-day cognitions and possible core beliefs or rules for living. These simple or mini formulations can be drawn out during therapy session discussions (see Figure 3.6) and can be a diagrammatical way of summarising a conversation. They can also be added together and developed further as therapy progresses and add to a fuller, more comprehensive formulation.

> **Example:** [Continuing with Marie.] Marie believes that she is worthless. She is embarrassed of her body, and does not want to go out in public. She thinks that people laugh at her and that she is unattractive.

Focusing on the relationship between different components of the model through a formulation can help the person to learn about key relationships and aspects that they are experiencing. Drawing out a formulation together during therapy can be a very collaborative process and can help the therapeutic relationship.

Three of the most common type of formulations used in CBT are: maintenance formulations, historical/longitudinal formulations, and problem-specific formulations.

> Historical/ longitudinal formulations dispel the myth that CBT ignores the past and only focuses on the here and now.

- *Maintenance* – these are ways of demonstrating how a difficult event or situation triggers thoughts, feelings, behaviour and physical symptoms.

They can be used to:

- o Demonstrate the different elements of CBT.
- o Describe the interaction between those elements.
- o Discuss individual elements in isolation.
- o Provide opportunity to discuss current problems and events in therapy.
- o Find themes, e.g. repeated patterns of thoughts and key triggers.

- *Historical* – these are also known as longitudinal formulations because they show how early experiences can contribute to current difficulties. They show how beliefs, perceptions and behaviours have developed. They may particularly highlight traumatic events, attachment experiences and the quality of early relationships. They require open and honest discussions, and should always be focused on what is important to the person, and may also include significant events, relationships and physical/mental health issues.
- *Problem-specific* – these can provide a useful structure and highlight specific cognitive processes and relationships that might be particularly relevant. These provide a specific framework for specific problems. They often draw upon research findings of patterns and links that are associated with particular difficulties. There are many examples of these available in core texts such as Wells (1997) and Morrison (1999).

## Cognitive and behavioural strategies

CBT should be tailored to the individual's needs and guided by the formulation that has been developed. A useful way to describe the strategies used in CBT is whether they are aimed at cognitive or behavioural symptoms. Behavioural approaches are often adopted earlier on in therapy, or often used for individuals experiencing low mood where volition and motivation may be lower. These should be implemented following a thorough assessment and formulation of the function of certain problematic behaviours. Either way, the goal is cognitive change through discussion and exploration. Learning new skills is an important part of CBT as it is hoped that the person adopts skills that they will take with them and apply after therapy has concluded. The strategies detailed in Table 3.2 can be discussed and tried out during session, then practised as homework tasks. This should support the person to overcome their difficulties, through new ways of thinking and behaving.

So there you have it, the basic but core elements of CBT, in a nutshell. Once the basic theory and techniques are understood, we can be confident and creative in applying them to a variety of mental health problems and distress. The ultimate aim of CBT is to empower

| | Cognitive strategies | Behavioural strategies |
|---|---|---|
| Purpose | To identify common ways of thinking and explore unhelpful cognitions. | To encourage or to reinforce behavioural change, which should facilitate cognitive change. |
| Example techniques | **Thought monitoring**<br>Recording frequent beliefs and images and recurring information processing problems. People may need a lot of practice and within session work to help them to identify key thoughts.<br>When regularly occurring negative automatic thoughts/beliefs (NATs) have been identified, the therapist can guide the person to identify 'deeper' beliefs or more core beliefs. Questions about the NATs could be asked, such as 'What would be the worst that could happen?', 'What does this belief say about you?' (This type of questioning is referred to as 'downward arrow technique').<br>**Thought evaluation**<br>Questioning the evidence and counter-evidence for beliefs and cognitions. As a follow-up, alternative explanations can be developed to counter the biases in thinking styles. Also, alternative thoughts based upon the evidence you have found can be generated Socratically. This can be used for both automatic thoughts and deeper beliefs.<br>**Finding alternative strategies**<br>Other 'cognitive' strategies can include:<br>• Techniques to alter attention.<br>• Techniques to develop new cognitive skills, for example:<br>o distraction.<br>o controlled worry periods. | **Activity monitoring**<br>This can be used to highlight the link between key situations, thoughts, feelings and behaviours.<br>It can also identify triggers for problems and patterns of behaviours.<br>It can be helpful to 'scale' or score the level of emotions in particular situations.<br>**Activity scheduling**<br>Detailing how a person is spending their time can be a useful way to identify pleasurable activities. These can then be increased to reduce distress.<br>**Exposure work**<br>Aimed at gradually mastering a problem, the primary method is to develop a 'hierarchy' of difficult situations, and conquer them one step at a time.<br>**Behavioural activation**<br>Scheduling activities to encourage people to approach the activities that they are currently avoiding and by focusing on the 'cognitions' that they are using to avoid activities (see Veale, 2008). |

**Table 3.2** CBT strategies

a person to make permanent changes in their life. Using this approach you can truly engage in a collaborative way of understanding and resolving problems.

## CASE STUDY

John, 58, was referred for assessment and therapy by his GP. He was described as experiencing a trauma reaction after an accident at work, which he had not been able to get over and had subsequently become low in mood. He had been unable to return to work. John had been married to Christine for many years, they had three adult children who all lived locally, but saw them infrequently. John initially attended with Christine but wanted to be seen alone.

During the first session, John described feeling very low, and doing little activity throughout the day. He said his life had been finished early, that he was 'useless' and 'on the scrap heap'. He felt there was nothing to do, or to look forward to. John had worked throughout his life as builder, often doing shift-work and long hours. He'd had a good social life, drinking and playing snooker, but was not engaging in any of these activities now. John felt that he had had many friends and acquaintances, but currently wasn't in touch with many of them. He had sustained some back and joint injuries following his accident, and never recovered, despite many operations and physiotherapy.

In the early sessions, John was encouraged to talk and express how he was feeling; he found this difficult initially as he was a private man, unaccustomed to talking about himself in this way. We began to draw out a maintenance formulation, as John was discussing some specific incidents that he felt demonstrated the essence of his concerns. As John spoke, the therapist guided him towards grouping different aspects of his experience within different 'systems':

| | |
|---|---|
| *Situation*: | Yesterday. Sitting at home. Should have been meeting an old friend in the pub. |
| *Thoughts*: | I can't be bothered. It's too hard. What the hell is wrong with you? |
| *Behaviour*: | Stays where he is. Avoids going out. Ignores the phone. |
| *Physiology*: | Agitated, can't sit still. |
| *Feelings*: | Annoyed, fed up, frustrated. |

After developing a few maintenance formulations, John and the therapist identified that John was regularly avoiding activities. He complained that he was not used to doing 'nothing' and that this frustrated him a lot. A home task was developed to record exactly how he was spending his time over a few of the days before the next session.[1] He also rated how he was feeling throughout that day. This activity monitoring confirmed to John that avoiding socialising and going out caused his mood to stay low or get lower, and that he was more frustrated because he did very little but wanted to do more. Behavioural activation was therefore suggested as a way to move forward with this. John identified activities that he wanted to do, and we graded these activities according to how achievable John felt they were. Home tasks included activity scheduling to keep a record of how he did, and thought monitoring.

After a few weeks of trying some graded activities (such as spending time in his 'local pub' and going to the betting shop), when discussing John's progress during sessions it was clear that specific thoughts were occurring such as 'I hate it here', 'I don't belong here anymore', 'I'm not the man I used to be', and that these activities were resulting in a dip in his mood. These were all beliefs that had been picked up in John's dialogue in the early sessions but the behavioural tasks were eliciting more thoughts about himself. This led to discussions in sessions about whether the activities were appropriate for John, did he still enjoy them? John acknowledged that they made him feel worse because they were activities he used to do when he was younger. He no longer wanted to be in those environments. An alternative list of activities was developed and subsequent behavioural tasks planned.

Dysfunctional thought records (DTRs) (Figure 3.7) were used to provide a structure to thought monitoring to enable John to develop his skills in accessing his cognitions. John gradually became more aware that he was having trouble accepting that his working life was now over. He was also having trouble accepting his current role in society and his physical problems. John was generating similar thoughts and beliefs earlier, but he had not made the link between these beliefs and how he was feeling. Socratic dialogue was used to explore the link that kept occurring in his thought records.

We then began to explore John's beliefs more, using a downward arrow technique to try to identify deeper beliefs:

*John*: I'm not the man I used to be.
*Therapist*: Why is that so difficult for you right now?
*John*: It means I can't do what I used to do.
*Therapist*: What does that mean about who you are now, John?
*John*: I'm not a 'man', I'm not me.
*Therapist*: What does that mean about you?
*John*: It means I'm pathetic, finished, useless ...

*(Continued)*

*(Continued)*

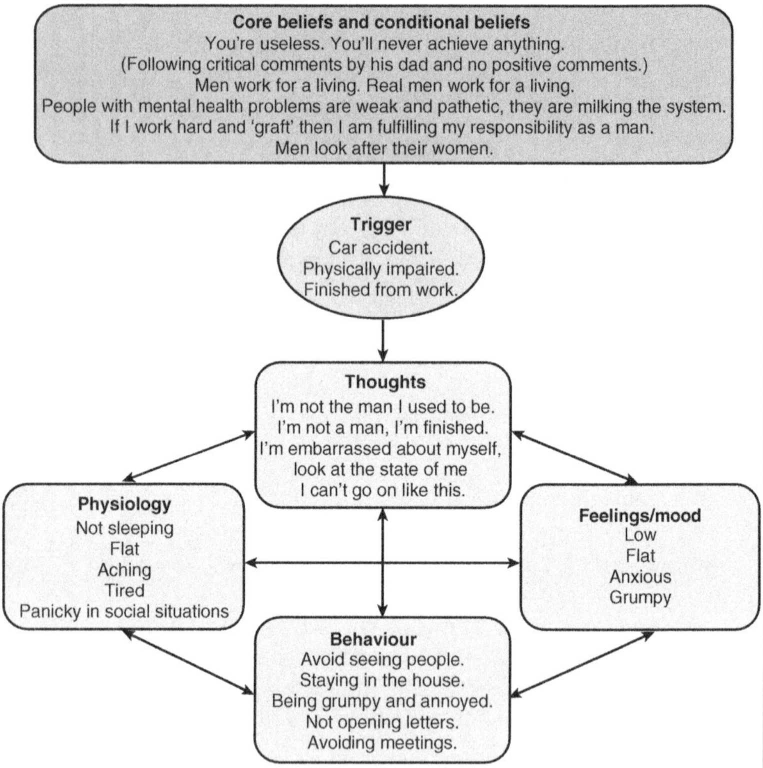


**Figure 3.7** Example of a case formulation

We then focused in on this final, key thought, and where it could have originated from. This led to discussions about John's childhood; his dad's critical management of John over his brothers; John's work ethic; and the fact that he used to believe that people with 'emotional' problems were 'weak, pathetic, and faking their problems'. Home tasks and discussions in sessions centred on gathering evidence around this belief. John initially gave lots of evidence for this, but moved on to providing clear examples that did not support the beliefs. Psychoeducation was also used to give John a full understanding of what depression was. After several more sessions, John was able to generate an 'alternative thought' around the idea that his life as a 'working man' was now over, but that this was no fault of his own. He acknowledged that he had to embrace a new way of living his life and 'adjust' to the changes. Behavioural tasks were set up that John was able to engage in more fully. He tried out new activities and rating how they made him feel.

When therapy ended, John had completed 15 therapy sessions. He was beginning to accept that he is now essentially a 'retired' man, and that this is an OK position to be in. He was changing his attitude towards mental health issues by further reading and research. John also attended a self-help group for individuals with mental health needs. He met some 'quite normal people'. John and his wife were beginning to get involved in activities that were more suited to his age and physical needs. He made a friend with similar needs whilst attending a swimming group for older adults. His mood was more positive and stable, and his sleep improved a little, which he felt was very beneficial for his overall functioning.

## NEW-WAVE CBT

CBT has developed in both theory and application. There are new and emerging ways of working under a CBT umbrella. Two of these are briefly summarised below.

### Metacognitive therapy

Metacognitive therapy (MCT) aims to modify the way in which thoughts are experienced and regulated. Metacognitions are defined as positive beliefs about the need to worry, ruminate or monitor stress. MCT – based on the self regulatory executive functioning model (S-REF model, Wells and Matthews, 1994) – suggests that problems are caused by the way thought processes are controlled and the styles:

- *Worry and rumination* – verbal thinking styles, which occur as an attempt to 'cope', but they act to prolong anxiety and negative affect by focusing an individual on certain cognitions and processes that strengthen problematic beliefs.
- *Threat monitoring* – attention is focused on sources of threat, internal and external, again as an attempt to cope or to help themselves, resulting in an increased awareness of threat and more problematic thoughts and negative emotions.
- *Avoidance and thought suppression* – strategies also adopted in an attempt to help, but they cause problems by failing to produce any evidence against the problematic thoughts.

Therapy therefore focuses on allowing people to experience different relationships with cognition and manipulation of cognitive processes used, such as worry. Techniques used are attention training, detached mindfulness and situation attentional refocusing. Techniques from CBT can be used but focusing on the metacognitive belief level, not the cognitive content.

### Acceptance and commitment therapy

Acceptance and commitment therapy (ACT) has been described as 'enriched CBT', and the origins are based in behavioural theory. The underlying idea is that a person's difficulties exist or are exacerbated because they are trying to control feelings and thoughts either by avoiding or escaping from them. The aim of ACT is to increase flexibility, and there are six core processes involved in this: 1. *Acceptance*, which is to accept and embrace problematic feelings with awareness rather than avoid them. 2. *Cognitive diffusion* is about being with a painful thought or feeling. The thought can be examined, reported, spoken out loud and experienced till it diminishes. 3. *Being in the present* and 4. *Understanding self in context* addresses how a person *is* in the present moment, experiencing the here and now rather than living in the mind, going over past or hypothetical future events. Mindfulness exercises and metaphor are used here. The last two are 'activation' processes aimed at helping the person to move forward: 5. *Clarifying and understanding core values* and 6. *Committing to action*.

## GLOSSARY

| | |
|---|---|
| Activity scheduling | Scheduling activities that may be found pleasurable or meaningful with the aim of breaking the vicious cycle between low mood and reduced activity. |
| Behavioural activation | Activity scheduling to encourage people to do activities that they are avoiding and analyse the cognitive processes (e.g. rumination) that serve as a form of avoidance. |
| Conditional beliefs | Also referred to as 'rules for living'. Beliefs that are usually expressed as if/then. The rationale of the belief is contingent on something else. |
| Controlled worry periods | A specific period of time in which the person 'allows' themselves to 'worry'. |
| Cognitions | Verbal events or images in the stream of consciousness. |
| Collaborative empiricism | *Collaborative*: Actively and deliberately interacting with the person, using skills to encourage the person to actively engage with their therapy. |

| | |
|---|---|
| | *Empiricism*: Using a 'scientific' stance in 'discovering' and evaluating cognitive processes. |
| Core beliefs | Deeply held beliefs. They are often basic and extreme and formed early on. |
| Directive | Psychotherapy whereby the therapist asks questions and can take the 'lead' of the therapeutic process. |
| Distraction | The deliberate diversion of the person's attention. |
| Dysfunctional thought records (DTR) | Worksheets designed to methodically gather information regarding thoughts that are problematic and distressing for an individual. |
| Five-systems model | It is thought that psychological problems occur from a combination of 'events' that are interrelated across five domains: thoughts, feelings, behaviour, physiology and what is going on in the environment (Greenberger and Padesky, 1995). |
| Formulation | A shared understanding of the person's problems. A way of applying psychological theory to the difficulties and experiences of others. |
| Home tasks | Also known as 'homework'. Tasks carried out at home between therapy sessions. Intended to discover new information relevant to the therapy or to reinforce skills being developed. |
| Guided discovery | Verbally guiding the person to 'discover' or become aware of information that is currently outside their awareness. |
| Longitudinal formulations | A shared understanding of a person's problems which explicitly acknowledges and incorporates early experiences and hypotheses about early core beliefs and conditional beliefs that may have developed and that may underpin current difficulties. |
| Psychoeducation | Factual-based information that is given to the person during the course of therapy, relevant to their presenting problems and symptoms. |
| Schema | A set of deeply held beliefs that produces a consistent way of thinking about self, others and the future. |
| Socratic dialogue | A form of dialogue and purposeful questioning that guides a person to discover (for themselves) overlooked information and links between events and occurrences. |

| | |
|---|---|
| Socratic questions | Types of questions that guide someone towards new information about themselves or makes links and discovers relationships between symptoms or events. |
| Socialisation | Orientating someone towards the 'cognitive model' of therapy. |
| Thought evaluation | Also known as thought 'challenging'. Guiding someone to evaluate the evidence that they base their beliefs upon. |

## REFERENCES

Beck, A.T., Rush, A.J., Shaw, B. F. and Emery, G. (1979) *Cognitive Therapy of Depression*. New York: Guilford Press.

Greenberger, D. and Padesky, C. (1995) *Mind Over Mood*. New York: Guilford Press.

Morrison, A. P. (1999) 'Cognitive behavioural therapy for psychotic symptoms in schizophrenia', in N. Tarrier, A. Wells and G. Haddock (eds), *Treating Complex Cases: The Cognitive Behavioural Therapy Approach* (pp. 195-216). Chichester: Wiley.

Padesky, C. (1993) 'Socratic questioning: Changing minds or guiding discovery?' A keynote address delivered at the European Congress of Behavioural and Cognitive Therapies, London, 24 September.

Veale, D. (2008) 'Behavioural activation for depression', *Advances in Psychiatric Treatment*, *14*, 29-36.

Waddington, L. (2002) 'The therapy relationship in cognitive therapy: A review', *Behavioural and Cognitive Psychotherapy*, *30*, 179-191.

Wells, A. (1997) *Cognitive Therapy for Anxiety Disorders: A Practice Manual and Conceptual Guide*. Chichester: Wiley.

Wells, A. and Matthews, G. (1994) *Attention and Emotion: A Clinical Perspective*. Hove: Erlbaum.

## FURTHER INTRODUCTORY READING

Grant, A., Townend, M., Mills, J. and Cockx, A. (2008) *Assessment and Case Formulation in Cognitive Behavioural Therapy*. London: Sage.

Grant, A., Townend, M., Mulhern, R. and Short, N. (2010) *Cognitive Behavioural Therapy in Mental Health Care* (2nd edn). London: Sage.

Westbrook, D., Kennerley, H. and Kirk, J. (2007) *An Introduction to Cognitive Behavioural Therapy: Skills and Application*. London: Sage.

## NOTE

1. A brief internet search will bring up many worksheets that can be helpful in this process or useful worksheets can be found in Greenberger and Padesky (1995).

# Worksheet 3.1

## Basic formulation

During discussions in early therapy sessions, information can be recorded under the headings below to guide what type of information is discussed and to begin to socialise the person to these aspects of therapy.

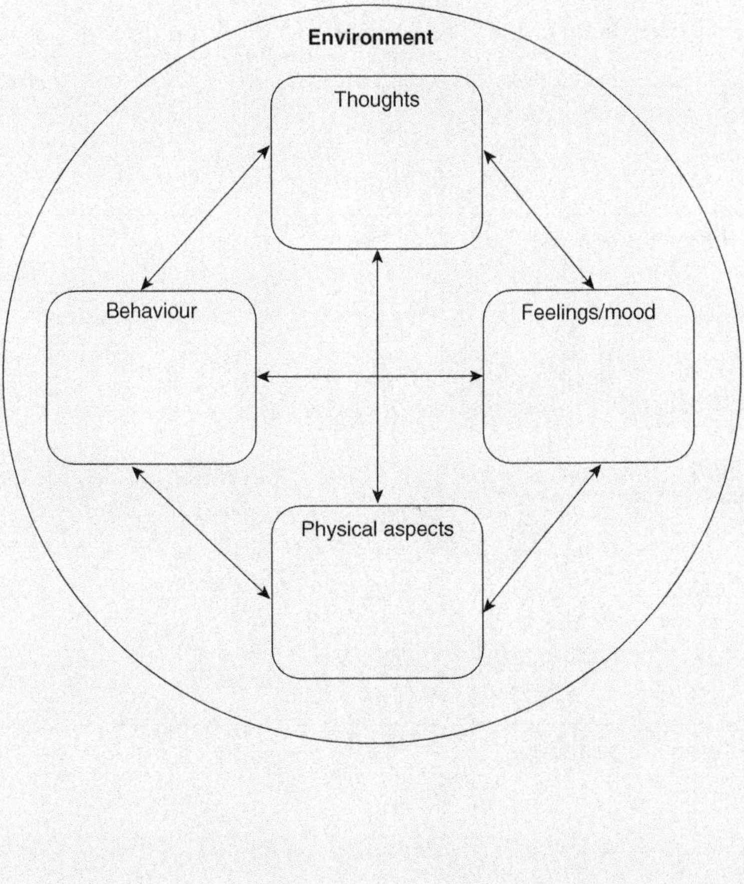

## Worksheet 3.2

## Thought diary

This worksheet can be used to allow discussion more fully around the cognitions and thoughts that the person is experiencing, and can begin the process of thought evaluation by gathering information about the evidence for and against the negative thoughts. Further discussion can then begin about an alternative thought. After being worked through within sessions, these sheets can be used for home tasks.

| | |
|---|---|
| Situation (environment) | |
| How were you feeling? | |
| What was going on in your head? | |
| Evidence for this thought | |
| Evidence that does not support this thought | |
| Alternative thought | |

## Worksheet 3.3

## Activity monitoring

| | Morning | Afternoon | Evening |
|---|---|---|---|
| Sunday | | | |
| Monday | | | |
| Tuesday | | | |
| Wednesday | | | |
| Thursday | | | |
| Friday | | | |
| Saturday | | | |

Activity monitoring can have a number of uses, including:

- Detailing how a person is spending their time.
- Identifying pleasurable and beneficial activities.
- Identifying activities that are not useful for that person.
- Scaling or scoring emotion ratings in specific situations and activities.
- Identifying triggers for problems.
- Identifying patterns of behaviour.
- Providing examples for formulation within sessions to enable links to be drawn between key situations, thoughts, feelings and behaviour.

# Worksheet 3.4

## Formulations in therapy

Formulations provide a shared understanding of the origins, development and ongoing maintenance of a person's problem. Formulations can be used within a therapy session to guide conversations and influence change. Here are some ideas on how you can use a formulation in the therapy session.

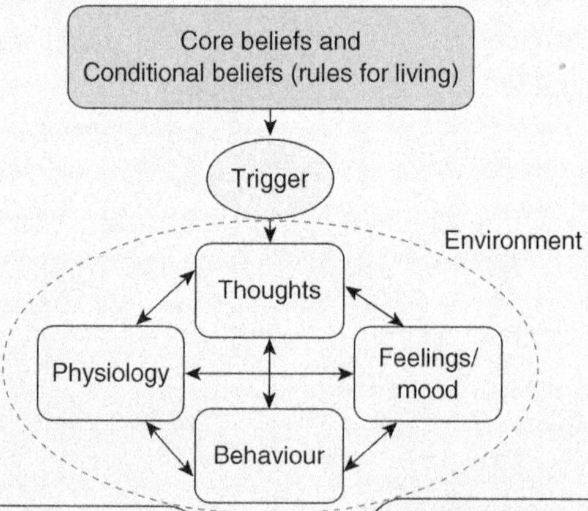


**Framing the problem**
Mapping out the effect of the problem can help the person realise how they may have become stuck in their current response.

**Spotting/managing trigger**
Ask the person to consider 'what situations typically cause the responses to occur'.These are then written in the trigger box.

**Links to core beliefs**
Once triggers have been spotted, ask the person to think about what is going on for them now and how this may have activated their core beliefs: how, why... long, etc.

**Framing improvement**
If the person provides an example of managing their problem effectively, ask 'which parts of our formulation were different in that situation, why?' Record these on the diagram.

**Where to start**
Ask the person to identify which parts of the formulation they want to focus on changing.

**Shoulds, musts and oughts**
Discuss what the person's common rules for living may be, in relation to their core beliefs.

# 4 COGNITIVE ANALYTIC THERAPY

Sharon Twigg

Cognitive analytic therapy (CAT) was developed in the late 1970s and can be applied within a number of different settings such as in groups, supervision, team work and individual therapy. CAT is a time-limited therapy that draws on the principles of cognitive and psychodynamic theory. This combined approach helps a person to think about themselves in terms of their thoughts, feelings and behaviours and how these components were and continue to be influenced by their early experiences of relationships and roles as a child. Exploration of learnt roles and patterns of behaviours are discussed in therapy to help a person understand their current difficulties or emotional challenges.

## THE MODEL

Cognitive analytic therapy (CAT) is an integrative model that went through a decade of evolution before first being put into practice in the 1990s. The driving force behind its development was a group of therapists in the 1980s (including Anthony Ryle) who set themselves the task to develop a therapy that covered three main goals:

1. To develop a therapy that could be effectively used within the British National Health Service.
2. To standardise the psycho-therapeutic approach and the language used by the approach.
3. To effectively contribute to therapy and therapeutic research.

> For a detailed account of the broad theoretical and philosophical writings underpinning CAT, have a read of Burkitt (1991), Ryle (1991, 1995) and Ryle and Kerr (2005).

CAT, as developed by Anthony Ryle and his colleagues, draws its grounding theory from psychological research and models, with an emphasis on cognitive and psychodynamic therapy. The CAT model is built on the premise that overcoming a problem requires a full understanding of its routes, which is facilitated by identifying two key features: *reciprocal roles* and *maladaptive behaviours*. Both are discussed below.

## Reciprocal roles

Reciprocal roles develop in childhood when a significant person (e.g. parent) interacts with the infant. The roles experienced in early childhood with our parents/caregivers become the adopted reciprocal roles we use as adults. All infants respond to their parent's interactions, which in turn influences their parent's behaviour/role. This to-and-fro interaction elicits a 'self' derived role (in the infant) and 'other' derived role (in the parent) during each interaction. The roles can be both positive and negative (maladaptive), as explained in Figure 4.1. With time, the repetition of these roles can lead to them becoming stable across settings.

| Examples of positive reciprocal roles | Examples of negative (maladaptive) reciprocal roles |
|---|---|
| Loving ⟷ Loved<br>Caring ⟷ Cared for<br>Attentive ⟷ Valued | Abuser ⟷ Abused<br>Aggressor ⟷ Victim<br>Sadistic ⟷ Masochist |

**Figure 4.1** Elements of positive and negative reciprocal roles

The dialogue used around children develops into an inner dialogue, which individuals cognitively 'hear' as adults. Some of these dialogues may be positive, helping us see ourselves as 'a good girl/boy', 'daddy's little soldier' or 'mummy's helper'. However, less helpful or abusive reciprocations may lead to negative internal dialogues such as 'cry-baby', 'clumsy oaf' or 'nothing but trouble'.

As the person grows into adulthood, they may seek the comfort of familiarity by unconsciously seeking social interactions that mimic earlier experiences. Those with positive childhood interactions will seek equally positive others, and may be equipped with social skills to do so. However, those with less positive childhood experiences may fall into familiar behaviour patterns that were useful in their childhood environment, but cause problems to be maintained in adulthood.

## Maladaptive behaviours

Behavioural patterns that no longer work in a person's favour and have become maladaptive are understood in CAT as target problem procedures (TPPs). TPPs are patterns of behaviour that are unconsciously played out to meet the person's needs or to avoid a core pain, but actually end up maintaining the problem. CAT mainly focuses on three types of TPPs: traps, dilemmas and snags (for some excellent examples, see Wilde-McCormick, 2008).

## Traps

Traps are behavioural patterns that create vicious circles and make the problem worse. The 'fear of hurting others' trap is a common example. Here, a person may choose to keep their feelings to themselves because they believe it will avoid hurting others. However, by not voicing their feelings, others are left to assume, guess and misunderstand. This may lead to disagreements, arguments and hurt for all involved, thus maintaining the trap with evidence of why they should keep their feelings to themselves (i.e. for fear of hurting others).

## Snags

Snags are behavioural patterns that stop us from getting where we want to be because of the excuses or assumed consequences we convince ourselves of. These may be the 'yeah-buts' in a person's life. For example, a person may wish to ask someone on a date but avoids doing so because they think 'Yeah-but they would never say yes'. This fear of rejection does not stop the day-dreams, but is a perceived snag leading to inaction.

Snags can also arise from others who do not want the person to change because of the impact it may have on their reciprocal role. For example, 'I would love to go to university, but it would upset my parents as I would not be close enough to be there for them if they needed me.' Another barrier to change may be that it could lead to some guilt. For example, 'If I did move away to go to university and my parents took ill from worry, I would feel so guilty for moving away and causing them so much stress.' This is because by changing the person may alter the reciprocal roles of others around them. As a result, the person is 'snagged' by the fear of change or consequence, which limits their opportunity for new experiences, success, change or pleasure.

## Dilemmas

Dilemmas are patterns of false choices, where a person may assume that they have only a limited number of options and that these options are equally weighed against them. These dilemmas tend to be 'either/or' or 'if/then' choices that are maladaptive. For example, 'Either I continue feeling angry about keeping my feelings to myself or I tell others, hurt their feelings and feel bad about it.' This may lead to 'If I hurt them they will hate me and then not want to spend time with me again.' Consequently, the person may feel that either choice leaves them equally defeated.

## The main principle of CAT

Now that we have an idea of the reciprocal roles and the target problem procedures involved with the model, we need to understand the main principles behind CAT before thinking about its application. There are three main principles in CAT, which are commonly referred to 'as the three Rs': *reformulation*, *recognition* and *revision*.

> In CAT a worksheet booklet called a *Psychotherapy File*, is often given at the start. It helps the person identify their difficulties. For further discussion, see Ryle and Kerr (2005) and Wilde-McCormick (2008).

1. **Reformulation:** This is an agreed and collaborative understanding (usually in a written or diagrammatic format) of the person's reciprocal roles, issues, behaviour patterns, experiences, relationships and feelings that will be reformulated throughout the therapy.
2. **Recognition:** Here, the people involved in therapy jointly identify the core pain or the main problem the person is experiencing (the target problem), as well as recognising the TPPs (remember them? – behaviour patterns) that are maintaining these difficulties.
3. **Revision:** This is where the therapist helps the person to identify and discuss alternatives to their choice of reciprocal roles, relationships and behaviours. The process is aimed at promoting positive change. Small behavioural 'experiments' may be tried out by the person to challenge assumptions or feared changes.These provide an opportunity for reflection and discussion. This revision of the original reformulation is therefore ongoing during therapy.The main aim is always to gain a shared understanding of the person's current difficulties and help them to see potential alternatives to previously undesirable set ways.

As reformulation in CAT is an ongoing process, many people still have issues to work on after therapy has concluded. However, they will hopefully have a better understanding of their difficulties and a bunch of tools to help them make more positive changes in their lives. So with that in mind, let's have a look at how to develop those tools and apply the CAT model to therapy.

## APPLICATION

CAT is usually conducted over a set number of sessions, therefore it is important for the therapist to clarify the expected time period of the therapy to prepare the person they are working with, for a time-limited input. Usually there are 16 sessions, but complex cases may require 24 sessions,

| Section | Session no. (approx.) | Therapy action |
|---|---|---|
| **Introductions** | 1 to 2 | • History taking.<br>• Current problems experienced.<br>• Other information (e.g. mood diary).<br>• Introduction of Psychotherapy File. |
| **Target problems** | 2 to 3 | • Discuss completed Psychotherapy File.<br>• Discuss target problems (TP) and core pain.<br>• Discuss target problem procedures (TPPs). |
| **Reformulation** | 4 | • Present reformulation letter and discuss with person. |
| **Developing the sequential diagrammatic reformulation** | 5 to 15 | • Develop the sequential diagrammatic reformulation (SDR).<br>• Continue process of reformulation, recognition and revision.<br>• Review person's week relative to TP, TPPs and SDR.<br>• Discuss alternatives and practical work.<br>• Discuss the meaning of ending for the person. |
| **Ending** | 16 | • Goodbye letter to person.<br>• Person's complete work folder (including reformulation letter, SDR, Psychotherapy File, etc).<br>• Letter to referrer summarising therapy and date of follow-up (copy to GP and person). |
| **Follow-up** | 2–3 months after ending | • Review person's progress.<br>• Evaluation.<br>• Further therapy?<br>• Write brief summary of follow-up session to referrer, GP and person. |

**Table 4.1** A typical 16-week CAT programme

while brief work may be conducted over four sessions. The process of a typical 16-week programme may look like the plan in Table 4.1, but as we are all aware, rarely does therapy follow a set program perfectly.

## Introductions

After reminding the person of the therapeutic plan, dates and times, the first meeting would be typical of most initial assessment sessions (e.g. history taking, current problems, person's expectations, person's diary log or mood diary). This usually involves discussions around the person's childhood, their relationships with parents/caregivers and other experiences that have had a significant impact on them. Examples of questions to get the 'ball rolling' may be:

- What are the memories that stand out for you when you think of your childhood?
- How would you describe the relationship you had with your mother/father?
- As a child, how did you overcome any difficulties you came across? Has that affected you now as an adult?

## Target problems

The aim of most therapies is to identify the target problem (or main underlying problem), and this is no different for CAT. This inevitably shapes the focus of therapy. Therefore, in the early sessions the person is asked to complete the standardised Psychotherapy File (Ryle and Kerr, 2005). In the beginning, target problems may be unclear or complex, so it is helpful for the therapist to clarify the details from the Psychotherapy File and ask further investigative questions or request examples. Typical target problems reported may be:

- I am unlovable and I don't deserve to be loved.
- I am a bad person who should never experience happiness.
- I can't forgive myself for being X, so why should anyone else.

Furthermore, the Psychotherapy File will help to identify the TPPs, which are the learned and repeated behaviour patterns that maintain the target problem. Further examples of dilemmas, traps or snags (as discussed previously) are:

- Either I am in control to keep things running perfectly but get tired, or I lose control and things go terribly wrong. (Dilemma)
- When I am down I believe I do things poorly and often end up making mistakes. So I question why bother? This leaves me feeling depressed, so I continue to make mistakes and feel low. (Trap)
- I would like close friends, but friends can be needy and want lots of time. So I put less effort into relationships, which maintains a 'safe' distance in my friendships. (Snag)

Identifying TPPs should help provide details of:

- What does a person do exactly?
- How do they view the world?
- When do things typically go wrong?
- Who responds/maintains the problem or maladaptive behaviour?
- Why it is repeated? What is the expectation of the person's actions?

Clear details at this point in the process should help a therapist understand why a person has come to therapy. This understanding will then be shared through a reformulation letter.

## Reformulation

By the fourth or fifth session, a reformulation letter is written (see the Case Study on pp. 66–71 for an example reformulation letter) which summarises the person's history and difficulties. Details should include:

- Current problems.
- Childhood experiences.
- Relationships and roles.
- Target problem.
- Target problem procedures.
- Self-evaluation.
- View of the world.
- Hopes for the future.

The reformulation letter is often read out to the person. This will be beneficial for two reasons. First, it will resolve any hidden difficulties a person may have with their reading, such as eyesight problems, low ability or dyslexia. Second, a person can reflect upon their life experience as heard through another person. This in itself can be very cathartic for people, as it may be the first time that they have talked about their lives in detail and had it summarised for them. Therefore, as suggested by Ryle and Kerr (2005), it is important that a collaborative effort towards gaining accurate descriptions and understanding is followed by the therapist from the start. Indeed, using the person's own words, descriptions or phrases rather than the therapist's helps share this collaborative compilation of the letter.

## Developing the sequential diagrammatic reformulation

Following the reading of the reformulation letter, work begins on creating a diagram of the problems and problematic behaviours. This is the beginning of what is referred to as an initial 'sequential diagrammatic reformulation' (SDR). This diagram visually represents the person's target problems, target problem procedures and reciprocal roles.

The use of having such a diagram in addition to the reformulation letter is that there is often too much detail or complexity in the verbal description alone. Therefore, a diagram aims to simplify and identify inter-relations between different problems that may not be obvious in the letter. It also allows a person to focus on their difficulties in an abstract way and to survey the various component parts of their target problem.

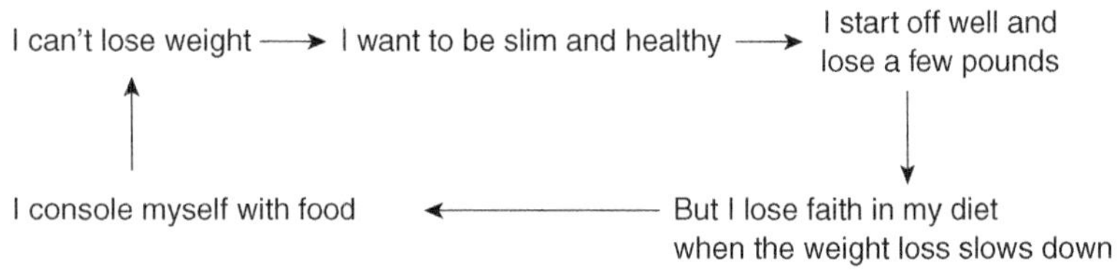


**Figure 4.2** Example of a common snag

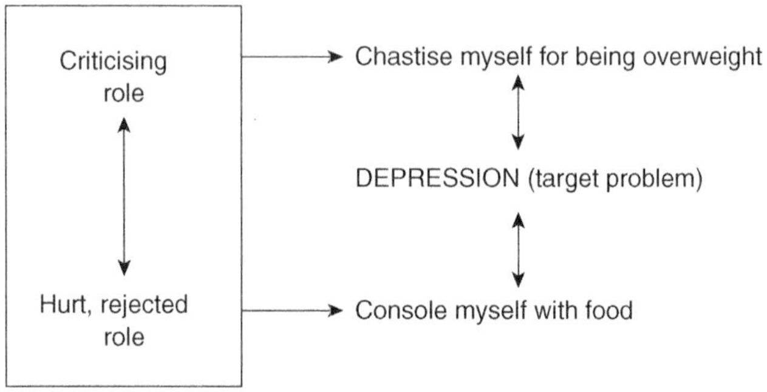


**Figure 4.3** Example of a single reciprocal role

The shapes of these diagrams are entirely different for each person, but each typically starts with a basic flow diagram which describes behavioural sequences (i.e. traps, dilemmas or snags), such as shown in Figure 4.2.

Further discussions provide additional details to the diagrams. Core reciprocal roles derived from childhood which are repeated in adulthood will also be revealed. Depending on the complexity of the reciprocal roles, single (see Figure 4.3) or multiple roles may be added to the diagram.

> Further issues of transference and counter-transference may also be identified at these points of therapy and should be discussed in supervision.

Throughout each stage of the SDR, the person will be asked to reflect upon any thoughts, feelings or changes that need to be made. This, once again, will tweak the accuracy and collaborative understanding of the issues. However, it should be noted that it is only human for a therapist to make mistakes or misunderstand a person's experience from time to time. Therefore, adjustments to the reformulation letter or SDR are normal and part of the 'reformulation, recognition and revision' process.

## Recognition and changes

Through the process of therapy, the therapist never aims to solve the person's problems but instead helps to increase their awareness and recognition of their maladaptive patterns that maintain their difficulties. For example, a person who could only focus on complaining about her husband was asked 'What might it feel like to be a friend listening to your complaints about your husband?'

With this reflection she began to see that this was not a good topic to continuously talk about in relation to her goal, to get closer to her friends. She then identified her maladaptive pattern 'to share her feelings with others so completely' as sabotaging her goal to make close friendships. Instead, lighter conversations were used in social situations, which improved her relationships greatly.

With recognition, it is hoped that a person can regain a sense of control over their lives and become aware of alternative choices to their present situation. People may then feel more able to make changes in areas of their lives where they are confident to start. Alternatively, people may choose to maintain their current situation, but feel a sense of a better understanding of their difficulties.

Those who wish to make changes may be encouraged to challenge their maladaptive patterns by trying alternatives. However, it is important to discuss these potential changes in therapy to assess any potential risk issues. For example, shouting back at a domineering boss may be an alternative to a passive reciprocal role, but the dangers may be that a person could lose their job.

## Ending

As the number of sessions draw closer to the end, it is advisable to talk sooner rather than later about what ending therapy will mean for the person accessing therapy. Endings discussed in the person's history and their view of the world will help gauge how well they are likely to cope (Sanders and Willis, 2005). This will help the therapist prepare the person as an ending draws near, and reduce the chance of a negative experience when it eventually happens, for example: 'Well Stacey, we have six sessions left of therapy and I'm wondering how you feel as we draw closer to an ending?'

In the final sessions, the person is provided with a closure to therapy and time to reflect on the work conducted. The therapist facilitates this through a 'goodbye' letter, which summarises the changes that have happened since the start of therapy. This letter is read aloud to the person, highlighting the tools, resources (e.g. friends and family) and strengths a person can use to continue their progress, for example: 'Although this last session may seem like an ending to your therapy, I think we both recognised how many new options you have ahead of you. With the help of your friends and family you told me you felt hopeful towards fulfilling your life-goal of becoming a teacher. With the college resources and the work experiences you have completed, you told me how much more confident you feel in your ability now that you can 'hear' praise without it being silenced by the voice of doubt.'

People who struggle with endings may appreciate the opportunity to write a 'goodbye' letter to the therapist. This may provide a positive experience as well as to formalise the therapeutic ending. It may also provide the opportunity for the person to voice their feelings towards the process and their journey through therapy.

## Follow-up

All the potential changes are seldom completed by the end of the therapy. However, the CAT model simply aims to provide a person with the materials they can use to continue their progress, rather than to solve their problems. For this reason, most people are offered a follow-up appointment two to three months after therapy has ended, to discuss the continued process, evaluate the experience and reflect upon the initial patterns identified at the beginning of therapy. Further therapy may also be decided upon at this point and discussed with the person.

### CASE STUDY

Louisa, a 29-year-old female, was struggling to engage with her husband and two children because of her clinical depression and anxiety. After an initial assessment session, she was offered a 16-session plan of CAT.

Early discussions of Louisa's childhood revealed she was born following her parent's separation and her father remained an unspoken figure in her life. Further discussions revealed Louisa's mother as being angry, critical, rejecting and controlling. This often left Louisa feeling hurt, unlovable, needy and rejected during her childhood. Over time, the roles reciprocated between Louisa and her mother became part of her state of being, and engaged during social interactions (see Figure 4.4).

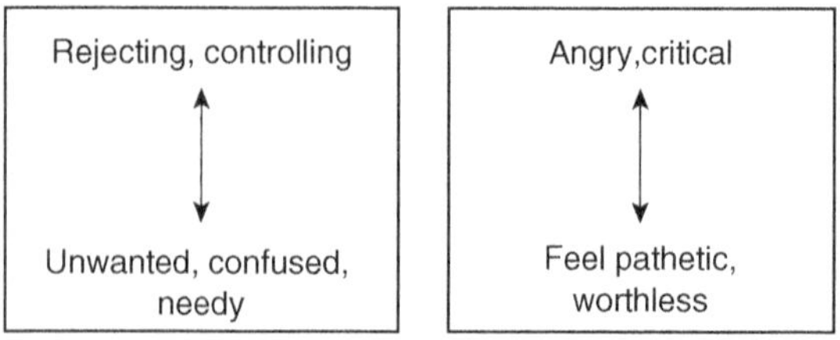


**Figure 4.4** Reciprocal reactions between Louisa and her mother

## Identifying the target problem procedures

The Psychotherapy File highlighted a number of traps, dilemmas and snags for Louisa, but three main target problem procedures were identified as:

1. **Trap:** The fear of hurting others and sounding critical like mum means that I do not express my true feelings. This helps me keep my promise to not hurt people, but leaves me feeling angry or my feelings 'brushed off' by others. It also means I sometimes choose to keep a distance from others to protect them from getting hurt.
2. **Dilemma:** Believing that other people's needs are more important than my own means that I try to satisfy other's needs without considering my own. While this makes other people happy and helps me feel 'good', I am left feeling worthless, but always striving to be valued. This often happens when my needs or feeling are overlooked, which leaves me feeling angry.
3. **Snag:** Telling myself I am a 'bad girl' like mum used to say leaves me feeling like there is nothing likeable about me. Then when I hurt people or sound critical I feel I cannot trust myself, so I avoid social contact. This leaves me feeling under-confident and anxious around people, so I try whenever I can to keep myself 'safe' by staying away from people by 'locking myself away' in my home. This leaves me feeling isolated, lonely and sad.

During the fifth therapy session a reformulation letter was read aloud to Lousia (Figure 4.5)

Dear Louisa,

Here is a summary of my understanding of what we have talked about in the recent sessions. Together, after our reading, we will discuss any aspects that you might feel helpful to talk about.

Louisa, you came to therapy feeling 'at your lowest point' with depression and anxiety. You told me how you always felt 'on your guard', or expecting the worst to happen. Social situations had become a struggle for you, so you avoided them altogether and chose to stay at home when you could. Often, this left you feeling guilty or lonely for ignoring your friends and limited the activities you could do with your children.

We started our sessions by talking about your childhood and you told me of your unhappiness from a very young age. You recalled that you were born following your parent's separation and your father remained an unspoken figure in your life.

*(Continued)*

*(Continued)*

You described the relationship with your mother as 'critical' and 'controlling'. You remembered constantly trying to do things right to please your mother, but always getting things wrong. Friendships also seemed to mimic this expectation and you recalled feeling torn as a child between different people.

On rare occasions you experienced happiness when your mother expressed how pleased she was with you, but your mother's pleasant periods were often short-lived. Another happy time was settling down with your husband and being overjoyed with the news that you were pregnant.

However, the birth of your baby was a traumatic experience that you believe left you with post-natal depression, which then led into long-term depression. Feelings of anxiety during social occasions also grew so unbearable that you avoided leaving your home.

I wonder, Louisa, if you learned from an early age not to expect unconditional love from your mother and accepted that it was your role to make her happy. It would seem that this expectation extended into other relationships in your adult life. However, this selfless role seems to come at the cost of neglecting your own needs and feelings. It also leaves you feeling angry and lonely when others fail to recognise your needs.

When you do express your feelings, it often comes out 'too raw' and angry, which leaves you feeling critical like your mother. This often leaves you feeling guilty and goes against the promise you made to yourself that you should never hurt others.

You recognised in your Psychotherapy File feelings of low self-worth and the neglect of your own rights as a person. I wonder if maybe your mother's indifference to your emotional needs has left you to also overlook this area?

Understandably, you have learnt to cope using ways which may have once been helpful, but have now become problematic. These areas are:

- To avoid hurting others and sounding critical like your mum.
- To meet other's needs before your own.
- To believe 'I am a bad girl' and do not deserve happiness.

During our therapy together I wonder, Louisa, if feelings of rejection or feeling criticised will present themselves and how we can work this out. Despite how uncomfortable these feelings may seem we must try to be aware of them and resolve them should they arise. I believe that working together for 16 sessions will provide you with enough support to begin exploring some of these difficulties and help you understand some of your fears.

**Figure 4.5** Reformulation letter from therapist to Louisa

**Drawing the SDR**

Once the main target problem procedures were identified, the SDR was drawn (Figure 4.6). Current examples of difficulties experienced each week in the 'real world' were added to the diagram. This helped Louisa recognise the reciprocal roles she adopted and the behaviour patterns she used to maintain her difficulty. This meant that Louisa could at times feel as if she was rejecting and controlling (like her mother), while at other times she would feel unwanted (as she felt as a child) in a number of social interactions.

In addition, the drawing of the SDR helped Louisa identify alternatives to her learnt patterns of behaviour. This often meant Louisa challenging her beliefs that: a) she should never hurt anyone, b) that other's needs were more important than her own and c) that she was a 'bad girl'. Alternative beliefs became more realistic and effective. These alternatives became known as 'exits', or alternative 'ways out' and are linked with the SDR. Louisa read through these when she became stuck and needed to remind herself of alternative choices. Exits for TPP 1 can be seen below:

Target Problem Procedure 1: The fear of hurting others and sounding critical like mum

Exits:

- This way of being helped you as a child to avoid upsetting your mother, but now this rule is no longer helpful as an adult. It is also inevitable to hurt people's feelings from time-to-time, but talking through such issues helps bring people closer together.
- Remind myself that keeping feelings to myself causes me much frustration and can be experienced as hurtful for others. Like everyone else, I can remind myself that I have a right to have an opinion even if it is different to others.
- It is OK to express my true feelings, including unhappiness, anger or dislike. I can use my assertive skills to express myself without sounding hurtful or critical. This allows me to be heard without sounding aggressive, but this will only come with practice.

With such exits, Louisa began to experiment with her social skills within therapy and finally in her life. Unsurprisingly, this helped Louisa enormously with her friends and family as they could finally start to understand her needs as well as share their own.

*(Continued)*

*(Continued)*

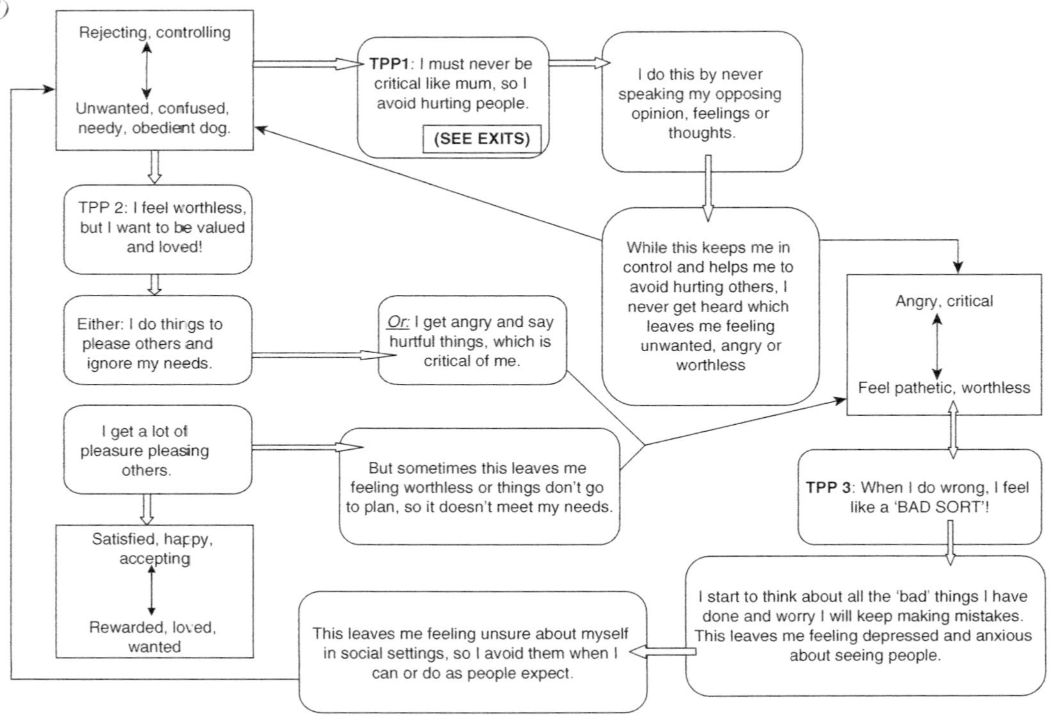


**Figure 4.6** Louisa's sequential diagrammatic reformulation (SDR)

By session 16, Louisa was aware that her therapy was coming to a close and a goodbye letter highlighting points of change and alternative life options was read to her.

Following therapy, Louisa began to recognise some characteristics in herself that went against the concept that she was a 'bad girl'. Talking to her friends, she found out that they valued her opinion and friendship. Furthermore, Louisa discovered by spending more time with her family that they enjoyed her company and that her children thought she was a good mum. Further on, she accessed workshops to help her with her assertiveness and social skills, which helped to reduce her anxiety.

## GLOSSARY

| | |
|---|---|
| Dilemma | False choices with limited options that are maladaptive and limit development. |
| Maladaptive behaviour | A behaviour that has been learned in order to survive in a given situation, but is ultimately negative and unhelpful when applied more broadly. |
| Reciprocal role | The role-related responses learned and developed in our early childhood that are used in relationships today. |
| Recognition | When the therapist and person jointly identify the main target problem. |
| Reformulation | An agreed and collaborative understanding of a person's experience in the form of a formulation (usually in a written or diagrammatic format). |
| Revision | The therapist helps a person to identify and discuss alternatives to a person's target problem procedures. |
| SDR | Sequential diagrammatic reformulation: an illustrated format of reformulation. |
| Snag | Behavioural act/response that stops us from getting where we want to be because of the excuses or assumed consequences we convince ourselves of. |
| Target problem (TP) | The main problem that is the focus of the therapy. |
| Target problem procedure (TPP) | The maladaptive behaviour and response that maintain the target problem. |
| Trap | Behavioural act/response that maintains the target problem or makes it worse. |

## REFERENCES

Burkitt, I. (1991) *Social Selves: Theories of the Social Formulation of Personality*. London: Sage.

Ryle, A. (1991) 'Object relations theory and active theory: A proposed link by way of the procedural sequence model', *British Journal of Medical Psychology*, *64*, 307–316.

Ryle, A. (1995) *Cognitive Analytic Therapy: Developments in Theory and Practice*. Chichester: Wiley.

Ryle, A. and Kerr, I. (2005) *Introducing Cognitive Analytic Therapy: Principles and Practice*. Chichester: Wiley.

Sanders, D. and Willis, F. (2005) *Cognitive Therapy: An Introduction* (2nd edn). London: Sage.

Wilde-McCormick, E. (2008) *Change for the Better: Self-help Through Practical Psychotherapy* (3rd edn). London: Sage.

## FURTHER INTRODUCTORY READING

Cowmeadow, P. (1994) 'Deliberate self-harm and cognitive analytic therapy', *International Journal of Short-term Psychotherapy*, *9*, 135–150.

Hepple, J. and Sutton, L. (2004) *Cognitive Analytical Therapy: A New Perspective on Old Age*. London: Brunner-Routledge.

Kerr, I. (1999) 'Cognitive analytic therapy for borderline personality disorder in the context of a community mental health team: Individual and organisational psychodynamic implications', *British Journal of Psychotherapy*, *15*, 425–437.

Pollock, P. (2001) *Cognitive Analytic Therapy for Adult Survivors of Child Abuse: Approaches to Treatment and Case Management*. Chichester: Wiley.

Pollock, P., Stowell-Smith, M. and Gopfert, M. (2006) *Cognitive Analytical Therapy for Offenders*. London: Routledge.

Ryle, A. (1997) *Cognitive Analytic Therapy and Borderline Personality Disorder: The Model and the Method*. Chichester: Wiley.

## ONLINE RESOURCES AND TRAINING INFORMATION

Association for Cognitive Analytic Therapy: www.acat.me.uk

# Worksheet 4.1

## Reciprocal roles

Here are a few examples of reciprocal roles found in different relationships. Some Roles can be positive and healthy like those seen in example 1, while others are adverse and damaging (examples 2–5)

**1. Typical parent-child reciprocal roles:**

| | | | |
|---|---|---|---|
| Loving | Caring | Protective | Attentive |
| ↕ | ↕ | ↕ | ↕ |
| Loved | Nurtured | Secure/safe | Valued |

**2. Adverse parent-child reciprocal roles:**

| | | | |
|---|---|---|---|
| Blaming | Neglecting | Fretful | Controlling |
| ↕ | ↕ | ↕ | ↙↘ |
| Guilty | Unwanted | Wary | Restrained Unruly |

**3. Adverse partner/relationship reciprocal roles:**

| | | | |
|---|---|---|---|
| Too loving | Abuser | Needy | Withdrawn |
| ↕ | ↕ | ↕ | ↕ |
| Smothered | Victim | Overwhelmed | Rejected |

**4. Adverse employer-employee reciprocal roles:**

| | | | |
|---|---|---|---|
| Demanding | Unappreciative | Critical | Unsupportive |
| ↕ | ↕ | ↕ | ↕ |
| Overworked/ stressed out | Under valued | De-skilled/ inadequate | Angry |

**5. Adverse therapist-person reciprocal roles:**

| | | | |
|---|---|---|---|
| All knowing | Interrogator | Inappropriate | Vague |
| ↕ | ↕ | ↕ | ↕ |
| De-skilled/ dependant | Interrogated/ Powerless | Vulnerable/ Wary | Clueless/ Unsupported |

# Worksheet 4.2

## Traps, snags and dilemmas

**Example of dilemmas:**

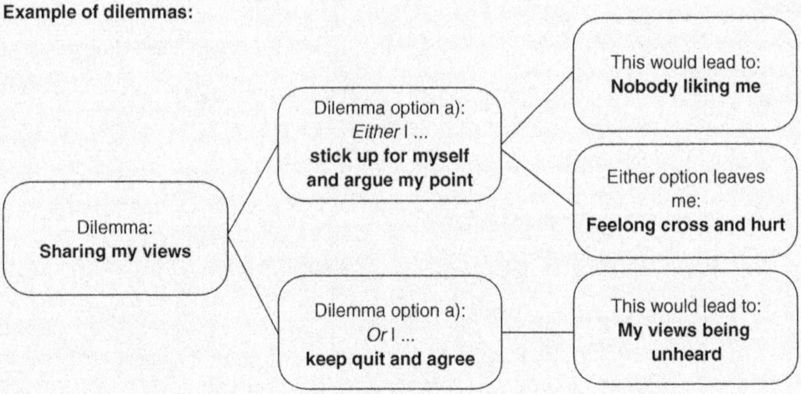


**Example of traps:**

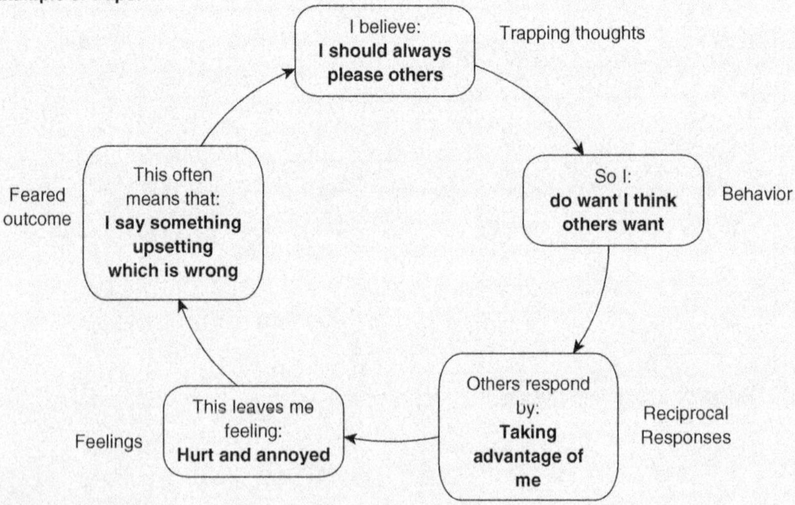


**Example of snags:**

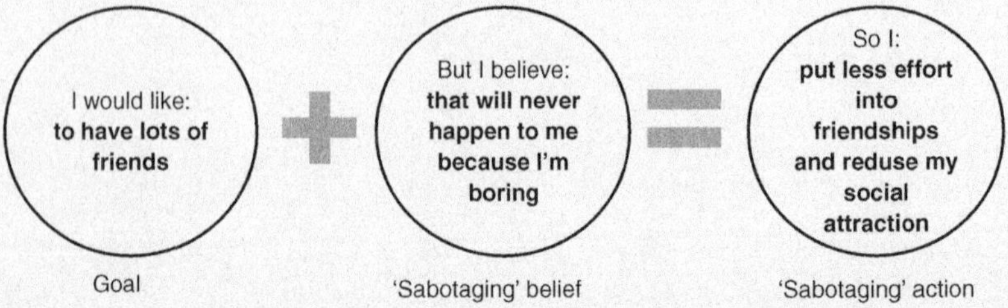

# Worksheet 4.3

## Basic checklist for therapists

| | | |
|---|---|---|
| **Session 1:** | Give person the Psychotherapy File (date__________) | (Yes/No) |
| **Session 2:** | Received Psychotherapy File | (Yes/No) |
| **Session 3:** | Review Psychotherapy File and discuss list of TPs | (Yes/No) |
| | Create reformulation letter | (Yes/No) |
| | Create summary list of TPs and TPPs | (Yes/No) |
| **Session 4:** | Read reformulation letter and TP/TPP list to person | (Yes/No) |
| **Session 5:** | Review person's week relative to TP/TPPs | (Yes/No) |
| | Create sequential diagrammatic reformulation | (Yes/No) |
| **Session 6–15:** | Discuss SDR with person | (Yes/No) |
| | Review person's weekly experience relative to SDR and TP/TPPs | (Yes/No) |
| | Begin to discuss meaning of ending | (Yes/No) |
| | Create goodbye letter | (Yes/No) |
| **Session 16:** | Read goodbye letter to person | (Yes/No) |
| | Receive person's goodbye letter | (Yes/No) |
| | Review meaning of ending and therapeutic experience | (Yes/No) |
| | Provide a follow-up date for person | (Yes/No) |
| | Write summary letter to GP, referrer and person | (Yes/No) |

# Worksheet 4.4

## Reformulation letters

When writing a reformulation letter, the therapist should use his or her, own words to ensure that the content is meaningful to the person accessing therapy. Below are some prompting points to help structure a reformulation letter.

| Points to consider | Prompts for therapist |
|---|---|
| Introducing the purpose of the letter | • To reflect on therapy sessions so far.<br>• To share your understanding of the conversations in therapy to date.<br>• Prepare for the work in future sessions. |
| What brought the person to therapy | • Why did they choose to come to therapy at this time in their life?<br>• Past and/or present difficulties that led the person to access therapy.<br>• Feelings the person was experiencing in day-to-day life when they came to therapy. |
| Life experiences that have contributed to the problem | • Any significant childhood or early life experiences reported in therapy?<br>• What were the relationships with family and friends like when growing up? |
| Feelings and behaviours that arose from life experiences | • What feelings did the person experience in light of their life experiences?<br>• How has this led the person to view him or herself?<br>• How did they respond, cope and learn to behave from these experiences?<br>• Has this led to any patters of behaviours in general life (examples)? |
| Formulating the persons experiences in the CAT model | • Explicitly questioning whether the person's childhood experiences could have influenced their current behaviours.<br>• How does this relate to reciprocal roles (i.e. how does their inner adult role reciporate the inner child role and visa versa)? |
| Naming the potential for process issues | • How might the self states and reciprocal roles play out in the therapeutic relationship?<br>• How will you both address these issues? |
| Plan for future session | • Understanding the reciprocal roles in more depth.<br>• Use diagrams to help summarise the connections between feelings and behaviours in relationships.<br>• Help to find ways of coping for the problem they described as (their language). |

# 5 PSYCHODYNAMIC THERAPY

Amie Smith and Kara Garforth

Psychodynamic therapy is one of the oldest models of therapy with its roots dating back to the late nineteenth century and the work of Sigmund Freud. Since then psychodynamic theory has evolved, resulting in different definitions of the key concepts. However, a fundamental commonality of all psychodynamic theories and therapies is the idea that people have an individual internal world. There is also general agreement that key concepts within psychodynamic approaches include the therapeutic relationship, boundaries, transference and countertransference, and the use of interpretation. There does, however, remain much debate about how these concepts should be applied to clinical practice.

## THE MODEL

Psychodynamic therapy is one of the many therapies derived from the psychoanalytic theoretical framework outlined in the work of Freud. This framework has evolved over the years, and several schools have emerged, each incorporating some elements of psychoanalysis and Freud's work.

Whereas traditional psychoanalysis involved in-depth, long-term therapy, often more than one session a week over several years, more recent approaches are briefer, time-limited (e.g. 16 sessions) and have a defined focus and limited goals (e.g. interpersonal psychotherapy).

> It is not possible to squeeze all the different theoretical schools of psychodynamic therapy into a pocket guide such as this. If you want to read more, see Lemma (2006) for an introductory summary, where, among other theories, you will see discussion of object relations theory. This approach, influenced by the work of British psychologists Ronald Fairbairn and Melanie Klein, focuses on relationships and how we are shaped by our early relationships.

The terms 'psychodynamic' and 'psychoanalytic' are often used interchangeably to refer to these approaches; however, throughout this chapter we will use the term 'psychodynamic'. There is a general consensus that the key concepts of the psychodynamic model are:

- the therapeutic relationship
- boundaries
- transference
- countertransference
- interpretations.

In this chapter we will offer our interpretation of each of these concepts.

The fundamental commonality that all psychodynamic therapies share is the importance placed on the internal world and the unconscious (things out of our conscious awareness). The process of becoming aware of aspects of ourselves that were previously out of conscious awareness is called 'insight', and you may often hear psychodynamic therapy referred to as an 'insight-orientated' therapy.

Psychodynamic therapy is based on the assumption that the symptoms a person presents with, such as anxiety or depression, are meaningful and are the expression of feelings that are out of conscious awareness. These feelings are out of conscious awareness because they are too painful to acknowledge and are in conflict with another perceived need. Therefore, expressing the feelings will result in negative consequences. Such painful hidden feelings are generally thought to have their origins in early life experiences.

> Freud initially proposed a model of the mind which identified three levels of consciousness, including consciousness (what we are aware of in the here and now), the preconscious (what is just out of our conscious awareness but that we can recall) and the unconscious (what is out of awareness).

We all develop ways to protect ourselves from painful feelings. These protective processes are also known as 'defences'; they include ways of seeing, thinking, feeling or behaving that serve to protect us from emotional pain or conflict. Given their protective role, it is important that the reasons for their existence are considered before offering therapy.

Defences are often repeated over time because they prove to be adaptive and continue to work well for us. However, these defences may become more harmful than helpful if relied upon over time, and in different circumstances to when they were first developed. Consequently, as our circumstances change they may cease to be adaptive.

**Example:** If in early life we experienced our caregivers as distant and disinterested, we may have developed defences that have led us to avoid talking to others about our painful feelings. Not talking to others may help us in the short-term, but we may continue to do this even when with people who are supportive and willing to listen. The defence of not talking to others about painful feelings may protect us from painful (hidden) feelings related to being let down by our early caregivers, but may in the long term be less adaptive.

Psychodynamic theory would suggest that the hidden feelings our defences serve to protect us from tend to find some means of expression, perhaps in the form of symptoms for which a person seeks help.

There is some debate about the aims of psychodynamic therapy, but it will usually focus on emotions, working with the person to help them bring their defences into conscious awareness. In turn, this can help them develop more effective strategies so they are able to cope with the feelings and live their life in a less painful way.

## APPLICATION

There is general agreement about the key components of psychodynamic therapy that facilitate the aims of therapy. Here, we offer our interpretation of how to apply these concepts to clinical practice.

### The therapeutic relationship

The relationship between the therapist and the person is considered to be one of the most important aspects of psychodynamic therapies. Although this is a fundamental aspect of all therapies, it is viewed as the vehicle for change in psychodynamic therapy, and it becomes the way in which painful feelings can be processed and dealt with (Lemma, 2006). Table 5.1 highlights and explains some key characteristics of the therapeutic relationship in psychodynamic therapy.

Because of the emphasis on the therapeutic relationships and interpersonal interactions, the people that find psychodynamic therapy most helpful are those who are able to recognise the relational aspect of their difficulties.

### Boundaries

The development of the therapeutic relationship is supported by the use of boundaries. Boundaries are the conditions or limits that are placed on therapy, which are viewed as an essential element of psychodynamic therapy. They serve to:

- Give consistency and predictability to the therapeutic space.
- Provide a secure base from which feelings can be shared, whatever those feelings may be.

| Key Characteristic | Explanation |
|---|---|
| Unconditional acceptance | The person is valued as a human being, no matter what their symptoms or problems. The aim is to allow the person to experience being accepted and not judged, which may be a new experience for them. |
| Neutrality | The therapist aims to remain anonymous. This means not sharing personal information, to allow the person to project, or put onto the therapist, feelings about themselves, their parents and other significant people. Projections provide the therapist with useful information about the person's other significant relationships and interpersonal interactions. The anonymous, neutral stance of the therapist can be mistaken for being aloof, distant and cold – common criticisms of this approach. However, this and all aspects of the therapeutic relationship are likely to be influenced by the individual style and personality of the therapist. |
| Containment | The relationship aims to be a holding environment or container where the person can express difficult emotions without the fear of the therapist responding negatively or rejecting them. This allows the person to experience a safe environment where they can explore and try out new ways of being, interacting and managing difficult feelings. This is sometimes referred to as providing a 'corrective emotional experience' (Lemma, 2006), where the therapist becomes a model of interpersonal relationships. |

**Table 5.1** Key characteristics of the therapeutic relationship

- Help the therapist gain a deeper understanding of the person, and their interpersonal interactions.
- Provide points for discussion, particularly when boundaries are broken.

Boundaries can be grouped into four types (Molnos, 1995), as explained in Table 5.2.

The breaking of any boundary is considered to be a communication of something, either conscious or unconscious. This will be discussed in the session with the aim of developing the person's and the therapist's understanding of their interpersonal interactions.

In setting these boundaries the therapist is similar to a parental or authority figure who sets limits. Therefore, having boundaries in place may evoke feelings for the person about these figures, even if the person's parents did not set boundaries. The feelings evoked can be both positive and negative and provide useful information about the person's past and present ways of relating to others. This can be talked about in the therapy session.

| | |
|---|---|
| 1. ***Place***: Sessions should take place in the same room, which will be laid out the same each session, e.g. the person and therapist will sit in the same seat each session. This helps to provide a familiar and safe environment. | 2. ***Time***: Sessions take place at the same time each week, on the same day of the week and for a fixed length of time (usually an hour). This helps to make the therapy predictable and consistent. |
| 3. ***Conduct required***: Both person and therapist are expected to start the session on time. The therapist and person will only talk and not offer practical advice – known as 'suspended action'. The aim is for the person to generate their own solutions through exploration of their feelings towards a situation. | 4. ***Relationship***: The therapist will maintain the boundaries of confidentiality and be honest yet not disclose personal information. The rationale for this is to not limit what the person feels able to talk about and express, e.g. if they know that the therapist is not religious, they may be more or less likely to express their own views about their faith. |

**Table 5.2** The four types of boundaries

## Transference

There are many definitions of 'transference', but the term broadly relates to the feelings that the person accessing therapy has about the therapist. Psychodynamic theory suggests that these feelings are transferred from other relationships and that this transferring of feelings is often outside of the person's conscious awareness. The person 'transfers', or 'projects', onto the therapist their own experiences of other significant relationships in their life, usually those of their parents. The effect of this is that the person's experiences of relationships will be mirrored in the relationship between them and the therapist. So what is happening in the therapy room tends to reflect what happens in relationships, current or past, outside the room.

> **Example:** A person may experience disappointment, confusion and anger with the therapist that may be similar to feelings they have towards an early caregiver. This is an example of negative transference.

Paying attention to transference can therefore assist the therapist in understanding the person's internal world and other interpersonal relationships in their external world.

Transference relationships can also be positive, where the therapist can be idealised by the person. Both positive and negative transference can be a risk to the therapeutic relationship if they are not understood and worked with.

The process of exploring the transference relationship is referred to as 'working in the transference' (Lemma, 2006). This process enables the person to

> Working in the transference is done through a process of making interpretations back to the person for exploration. These are referred to as 'transference interpretations'.

acknowledge the emotions and recognise that they are not personal to the therapist. This process is often done tentatively, at least initially, and does not always need to be done in reference to past relationships. During the early stages of therapy past relationships are not known, and so interpretations can only focus on the current relationship with the therapist.

**Example:** The therapist's hypothesis is that the person is feeling rejected by them and that the strength of these feelings is in some way related to (transferred from) another relationship. To help the person acknowledge transference feelings the therapist may say something like 'I wonder if you are feeling rejected by me'. If the person can recognise the emotion they may then be able to begin to work through the transference feelings in therapy sessions by tracing this emotion back to its root, which could be a relationship in the past, most likely a parent or sibling, or a relationship in the present.

> To practice from the psychodynamic model, therapists require knowledge of themselves as well as theoretical knowledge. For this reason therapists often undergo personal therapy to explore their own defences. Supervision is also essential, as it allows time and space outside of the therapy to acknowledge, process and understand the therapist's feelings.

Working in the transference needs to be done carefully and requires a degree of self-knowledge on the part of the therapist. It should also be acknowledged that the person and therapist also have a 'real' relationship that is not necessarily influenced by the past. It would be tempting to attribute all difficulties within the therapeutic relationship to the person's past experiences of relationships. However, the individual personality and communicative style of the therapist can influence the relationship they share with the person, and some of the person's responses are likely to be valid and appropriate to the situation and to what has been communicated by the therapist. So remember: not everything is transference.

## Countertransference

The feelings that the therapist experiences towards the person they are working with are referred to as the 'countertransference'. The feelings can be seen as an unconscious communication about the ways in which the person relates to themselves and others. It may be that we are experiencing feelings that the person is feeling, feelings that the person is struggling to express, and/or feelings that others may feel in relation to them. The emotions that are experienced by the therapist therefore give clues about how the person has experienced other relationships in their life and how they view the therapist.

Countertransference feelings need to be understood, worked through and used to the benefit of the person and therapeutic relationship. By asking ourselves 'Why do I have these feelings with this person at this particular moment?', we can seek to better understand the person. If the therapist does not pay attention to the reasons for the countertransference, they may respond in the way others have responded in the past, for example by 'acting out' aggressive feelings they have towards the person. This would result in patterns of behaviour being repeated, rather than being understood and offering the person the opportunity to explore a different way of being.

> When working from this model it is important to remember that therapists are human and the emotions we experience are also related to our own experiences of relationships. Just acknowledging our own feelings and protective process is often enough to not interfere with the therapy.

It is the therapist's responsibility to recognise countertransference feelings and prevent these from having a harmful impact on the therapy. This is where the therapist's knowledge of themselves and their defences comes in, so that they can separate those out and recognise the countertransference more readily (see Worksheet 5.3). Supervision is really important in helping you to do this.

## Interpretations

Interpretations are the therapist's way of helping the person to understand or gain insight into their difficulties, by making connections between their behaviour and their unconscious feelings. They link the person's internal experience with their external reality by putting into words the person's conscious and unconscious experiences.

Interpretations are considered to be an intervention in their own right, as they play a key role in facilitating the person's understanding and awareness of their difficulties. They also help to validate the person's experience of the therapy and demonstrate that the therapist has been listening attentively. It is a step beyond acknowledgement of the person's feelings. Interpretations are essentially hypotheses about the person's internal world which are to be tested out by the person.

Making interpretations is a difficult task and is a technique that is largely intuitive and which develops over time (Malan, 2007). See Worksheet 5.4 for more tips on making interpretations.

Having explored the key concepts, we will now consider how they fit into the three main stages of psychodynamic psychotherapy: assessment, formulation and endings.

## Assessment

The assessment process begins before the therapist has even met the person. They will look at the referral letter and any other available information prior to assessment to think about what is being communicated about the person:

- What is/is not being said?
- What is the tone/feel of the words?
- What is the relationship between the referrer and the person?
- What feelings does the therapist feel before meeting the person?

When meeting the person for the first time, it is important to consider the feelings – the countertransference – you experience throughout the sessions.

The assessment is often conducted over two or three sessions, with the first of these tending to be unstructured to allow people to bring what they want to talk about and describe their current difficulties. This also allows the therapist to observe how the person relates to their difficulties, and how they (the therapist) are related to this process. Further assessment sessions may be more structured, with the therapist asking more questions in order to gather information about the person's presenting problems.

> It is helpful to bear in mind that as the relationship develops and feels safer people, understandably, may feel more comfortable disclosing information and expressing their emotions.

The process of working in the transference therefore begins from the very first session, though initially transference interpretations will be made tentatively and perhaps without reference to the past.

In subsequent sessions the therapist will enquire about how the person experienced the previous sessions and whether they were able to reflect on the content and experience of the session, which is an important element of psychodynamic therapy.

The therapist may say something like 'The process of therapy can often evoke strong feelings, I wonder how you felt after the last session?' or 'What things did you think about from our last session?', 'How did you manage those feelings?', 'Is that how you would usually manage your emotions?'.

These questions will help the therapist to think about the suitability of psychodynamic therapy for each individual person, an important part of the assessment process (see Worksheet 5.1).

Some reasons why psychodynamic therapy may not be suitable include:

- *Anxiety* – the therapy may be too anxiety provoking, making it difficult for the person to honestly discuss and begin to face their distressing feelings. This is a common difficulty of therapy, particularly in the early stages as it is a new experience that is potentially very emotionally exposing for people.
- *Expectations* – psychodynamic therapy offers exploration and understanding rather than a directional 'how to' approach. If the person is seeking advice and instruction, then the psychodynamic approach is unlikely to be beneficial.

The psychodynamically informed assessment process also provides the person with a 'taste' of how the therapy is likely to be and helps them decide if it is for them; it may be that they feel other therapeutic approaches are more suited to them.

At the end of the assessment process the therapist will look for a way of organising and understanding the information in a way that is meaningful to the person. To do this the therapist will do a formulation, which informs whether or not the person will continue into therapy.

## Formulation

A psychodynamic formulation is an attempt by the therapist to explain how the person's problems have arisen and why they are continuing. A formulation aims to:

> If you would like to read more about psychodynamic formulations, see Leiper (2006).

- Account for the developmental origins of the person's difficulties.
- Account for the underlying conflicts and defences used to manage these difficulties.
- Highlight recurring interpersonal patterns and the person's expectations of others.
- Make predictions about whether change is likely and the possible consequences of change.
- Psychodynamic formulation is concerned with three elements, which Malan (2007) refers to as the 'triangle of conflict' (Figure 5.1).

'Hidden feelings' relates to those underlying emotions that are out of our conscious awareness. These are the feelings that underpin all of our behaviour and are generally thought to have arisen due to our early experiences.

**Example:** A person who experienced extreme criticism from their caregivers as a child may have hidden feelings of anger towards them. However, expressing these feelings would potentially have disastrous consequences, such as the withdrawal of care, which presents a conflict between other needs (i.e. the need to be cared for).

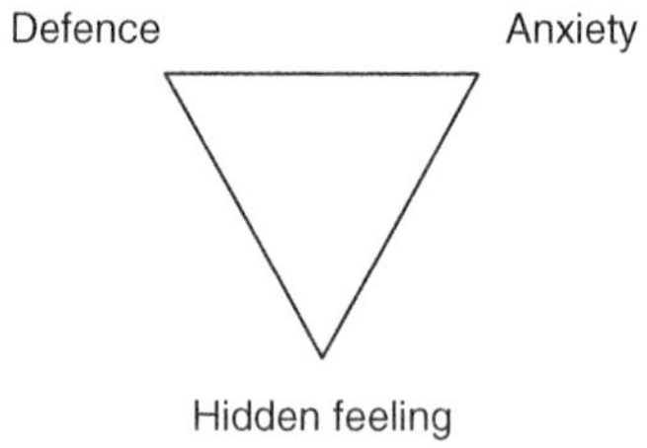


**Figure 5.1** The triangle of conflict

The triangle of conflict is presented this way (with the hidden feelings at the bottom) to illustrate that hidden feelings are less accessible in conscious awareness than anxieties and defences. The process of allowing the hidden feelings to emerge can take time, and it is important that this happens at the person's own pace. By the end of the assessment the therapist may have ideas about the hidden feelings that the person may not yet be ready to acknowledge. It is therefore important that the formulation at this stage only incorporates information, or interpretations, that have been made during the assessment. The process of the therapy will be to continue to explore the hidden feelings as they come into conscious awareness. Pushing the person to acknowledge feelings that they are not ready to face can result in them becoming overwhelmed and may result in them dropping out of the therapy.

The formulation will attempt to link the (hypothesised) hidden feelings to the *defence* and *anxiety* elements of the triangle to help the person to understand aspects of their behaviour as consequences of the hidden feelings, and ways of protecting themselves from those feelings.

*Anxiety* relates to the feared consequences of expressing the hidden feeling or impulse. Awareness of the hidden feeling causes anxiety because it is in conflict with another need, or an ideal that they hold in their conscious awareness, and so it has fearful consequences.

> **Example:** The individual with hidden feelings of anger towards his extremely critical caregivers fears that his need for love and care will not be met and that he will experience rejection or abandonment if the hidden feelings are expressed.

The anxiety feeling signals that there is something going on internally that threatens the state of being and the personality, so the internal world takes action to stop this threat by using '*defences*'.

Defences protect us from emotional pain by keeping the feelings out of conscious awareness or stopping the conscious mind acknowledging the conflict (see Figure 5.2; also Worksheet 5.3 for some examples). Because this process is out of our conscious awareness we are less able to adapt our behaviour to the external world and learn from our experiences to help protect us in the future.

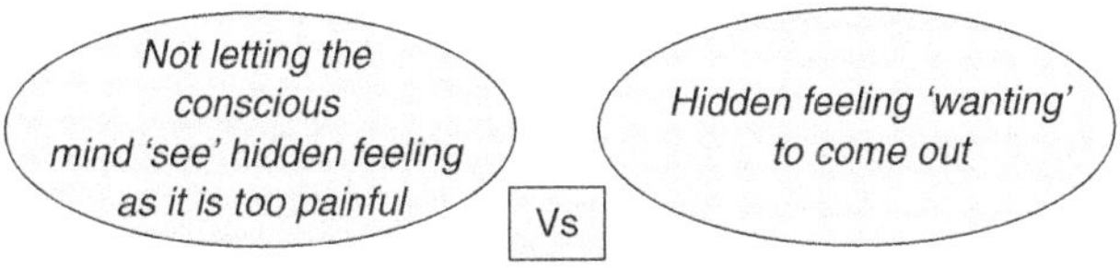


**Figure 5.2** The way defences work

So defences can become like a 'default button' in that the unhelpful patterns of behaviour are repeated. It is important, however, to consider that defences are usually developed for good reason, so they must be included in the formulation. The 'conflict' in the triangle of conflict therefore relates to the internal fight.

Once the therapist has developed an initial formulation they may share it with the person who has accessed therapy. The aim is to enable the person to begin to develop a new understanding of their behaviour, which they will build on over the course of the therapy. The intervention is similar in many ways to the assessment process; it is a deepening of the understanding they have achieved in relation to the elements of the formulation. As the therapeutic relationship develops, hopefully the person feels safer to acknowledge and explore more of their hidden feelings, bringing them into conscious awareness.

The main tool the therapist has is the use of interpretations to help the person understand their behaviour in relation to the formulation. These continue to help the person gain more insight into the relationship between their internal world and their external reality.

## Endings

Endings are particularly important in psychodynamic therapy. Most short-term psychodynamic therapies will work to an ending from the beginning. In practice this means that an end date will be set, and often the session number is explicitly stated week by week. Working in this way makes the boundary clear and allows the person to experience and work with endings.

> For more on the competencies associated with delivering psychodynamic therapies in clinical practice, see the competencies framework (Lemma et al., 2010).

The ending of therapy can evoke lots of powerful feelings for the person, often associated with loss as well as anxiety about separating from the therapist. The person has experienced the therapist as a 'container' for their distressing emotions for a period of time and the prospect of being without this can evoke strong feelings. An important part of the ending process is about facilitating the expression of those feelings, whether they are positive or sadness or anger.

The agreed ending should be stuck to and the therapist must be mindful of attempts to sabotage the ending.

**Example:** The person may present with more severe symptoms towards the end of therapy. This may be interpreted as an attempt to demonstrate their need for the therapist and a defence against the loss of support. The therapist aims to increase the person's confidence in their own ability to cope with the loss of the therapist and their feelings associated with the loss.

The therapist should be mindful of factors that may make the ending particularly difficult for individual persons, such as the experience of repeated rejections. Again, this should be discussed, encouraging the expression of their emotions and fears.

Endings can also evoke strong feelings for the therapist, which may vary across different therapeutic relationships. The ending could present as a loss for the therapist, though in other cases it may feel like a relief. It is important for the therapist to attend to their feelings about the endings and use these to inform their work. The therapist should be mindful of the transference relationship in the ending phase, as in any other phase.

**Example:** The therapist may experience feelings of failure at the end of therapy, which may be explained by the person's feelings about the therapy ending. The person may express that the therapy has not helped them, which may be a defence against the loss of the therapist. This could be interpreted to the person so that it can be discussed, increasing the chances of ending the therapy in a way that proves useful to the person.

So we have shared our understandings of the key concepts of the psychodynamic model and how they can be incorporated into the different stages of psychodynamic therapy. Much of the model is based around uncertainty, and takes a position of not knowing and of exploration. This means working with the uncertainty and being responsive to what the person brings. This can be really anxiety provoking initially, but it does get easier.

## CASE STUDY

Anna, aged 27, came to therapy because she was pulling her hair out, a difficulty she had experienced since childhood. She had recently had a baby and did not want her child to grow up seeing her do it.

### Assessment

#### *History of the presenting problem*

Anna first began to pull her hair out when she was 10 years old, when bullied at school. She kept it secret, except from family and close friends, because she worried what people would think. Anna was very self-conscious about it and spent time covering it up. She usually wore a hat, but during the assessment showed the therapist the extent of the hair pulling. The therapist's interpretation of this was that it offered a way of communicating feelings of shame and perhaps a way of testing out the therapist's reaction. Because this occurred early in the therapeutic relationship, these interpretations were not shared with Anna due to the therapist's uncertainty about her ability to tolerate them. Instead the therapist gently explored how Anna felt about others seeing her hair pulling, enabling her to acknowledge how it impacted on her feelings about herself.

Anna had tried many behavioural strategies to stop pulling her hair, such as wearing gloves, keeping her fingernails short and rewarding herself if she did not pull it, but she described the effects as limited.

### *Childhood experiences*

Anna was the eldest of three siblings and, because her parents worked, she was expected to care for her siblings and do housework. She tried hard to keep the house tidy in order to please her parents and continued to help out when she no longer lived there. Anna described her father as very critical of her, and said he never praised her, leaving her feeling 'not good enough', 'unloved', and confused about how to get love and affection. She described her mother as very passive, never standing up to her father.

### *Current relationships*

Anna described herself as a social person and the 'life and soul' of a party, though this did not reflect how she really felt. Since having her baby, she had begun to question the strength of some friendships and recognised she had tended to make more effort in friendships and often helped other people out. She felt disappointed that others had not offered support when she needed it. Anna acknowledged that perhaps she had done favours for others as a means of gaining praise and to be liked. She also acknowledged that she felt unable to talk to others about her emotions.

## Formulation

In the fourth session a verbal formulation was presented to her in the form of a therapeutic letter, which was read in the session. This initial formulation aimed to highlight the developmental origins of some of her emotions, such as feeling criticised and not being good enough. It also highlighted the function of some of her protective processes,

*(Continued)*

*(Continued)*

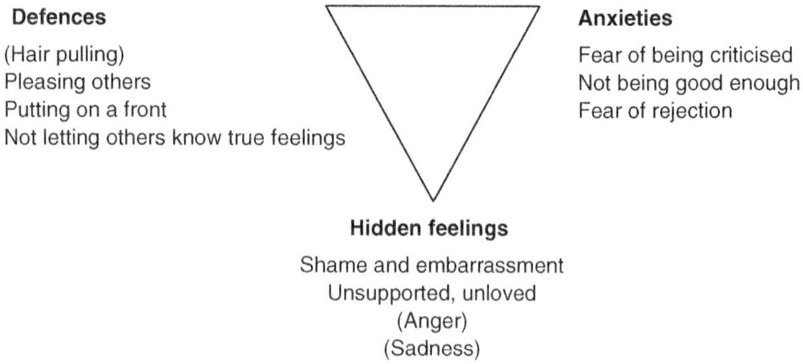


**Figure 5.3** Anna's formulation (after Malan, 2007)

such as pleasing others in order to not feel criticised and not good enough. A summary of the formulation is shown in Figure 5.3.

Anna had engaged well with the assessment, she had been reflective and willing to explore interpretations. She often found the process difficult, but was honest about this.

## Further therapy

It was agreed that a 16-session individual therapy, using a psychodynamic approach, would be beneficial. The therapy focused on building the formulation and supporting Anna to recognise the interpersonal aspects of her difficulties.

At times Anna looked to the therapist for practical solutions and instruction, which was discussed with her; she understood that psychodynamic therapy offered a process of exploration to identify underlying emotional difficulties that may contribute to her hair pulling. Anna's desire for instruction often left the therapist feeling not good enough. Through supervision these countertransference feelings were understood as being part transference and projective processes. Anna was perhaps seeing the therapist as like her father and was therefore expecting the therapist to respond in the same way (i.e. by telling her what to do). The therapist's feelings were therefore interpreted as part of the countertransference, and perhaps reflected how Anna felt when her father told her what to do. The relationship between Anna and the therapist was used to understand other interpersonal relationships.

Anna began to reflect on her interactions with her parents and recognised she helped out to try to please them. Over time she identified underlying emotional needs that were not being met, for example her need to be supported and cared for. Anna began to recognise times when she sought care and began to understand her own behaviour in a different way. For example, she noticed that getting distressed or 'creating a drama' was the only time her parents would take notice of her. However, she also became aware that it was after such occasions that she would pull her hair out. Anna began to understand her behaviour as a response to emotional distress and her needs not being met (i.e. not feeling loved and supported). Thus, she had increased awareness of the emotional needs underlying her behaviour and interpersonal interactions.

Through the use of interpretations and her reflections of her behaviour, Anna acknowledged painful emotions that she had previously been unaware of, such as feeling unloved, and also expressed anger towards her parents for not meeting her emotional needs. She recognised that the sensation of pulling her hair distracted her from this emotional pain and acknowledged this as a defence or protective process. However, Anna was able to recognise that the relief she felt was short-lived because she would experience pain, distress, shame and embarrassment about pulling her hair out. Anna was able to recognise this as a vicious circle. The more Anna saw the hair pulling as a means of coping, the more she felt she may not be ready to give it up.

**Ending**

Anna's goal was to stop pulling her hair completely. As the end of the therapy approached, Anna expressed disappointment that she hadn't stopped pulling. The therapist hypothesised that she was being experienced in the same way as Anna's parents, that is, not offering her what she felt she needed and therefore letting her down. This was discussed with her, allowing Anna to express her feelings of disappointment and sadness about the therapy and the therapist. In offering her a different emotional experience, Anna could acknowledge that feelings of sadness and anger could be tolerated, by her and by the therapist. Thus, the feelings were no longer hidden, and so were less painful and had less influence over her behaviour.

The end of the therapy was marked by another therapeutic letter that highlighted the new understanding of her hair pulling and as a reminder of the progress she had made. It also acknowledged Anna's feelings about the therapy ending

At the end of therapy Anna pulled her hair out much less and the area she pulled from was much smaller. She was able to recognise the progress she had made in understanding her interpersonal behaviour and felt she

*(Continued)*

*(Continued)*

was better able to manage her emotions. Anna was also able to express herself and get her needs met by asking for help when she needed it, rather than doing things for other people in order to get help. Anna observed that this resulted in different responses from others, particularly her parents.

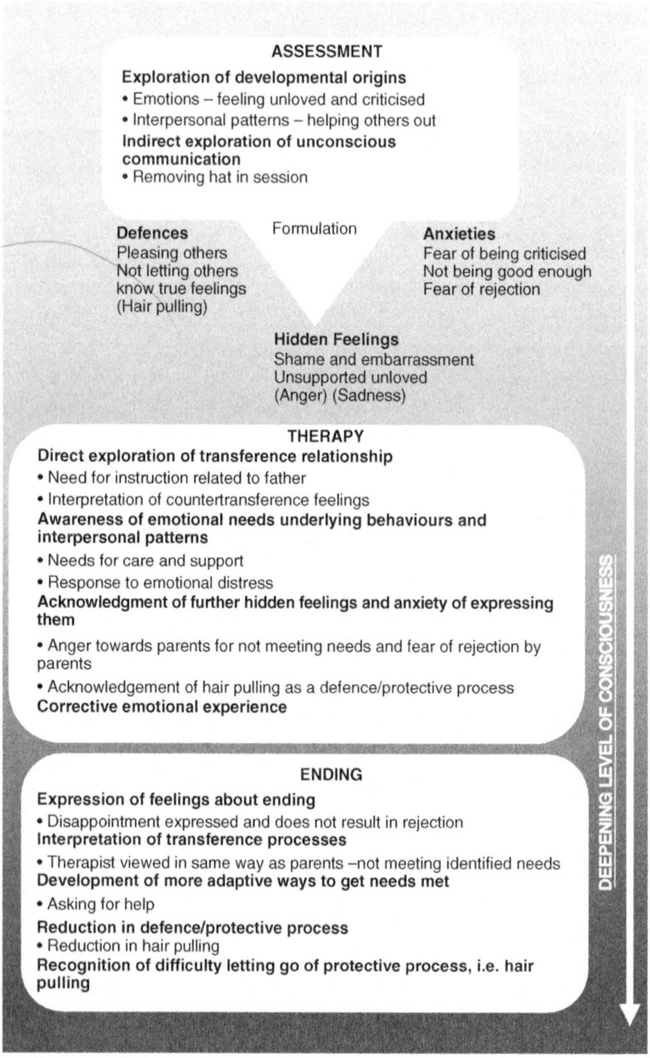


**Figure 5.4** Summary of Anna's therapy

## GLOSSARY

| | |
|---|---|
| Anxiety | The feared consequences of expressing painful emotions, e.g. expressing anger at unavailable caregivers may result in the loss of any love or affection, therefore the *anxiety* would be fear of rejection. |
| Boundaries | The conditions or limits that are placed on therapy, e.g. time: sessions take place at the same time each week. |
| Countertransference | The feelings that the therapist has in reaction to the person, some of which are transferred by the person, and reflect what the person feels about, or is doing to, the therapist. |
| Defences | The means by which humans keep painful emotions out of conscious awareness and protect themselves from pain. Also known as 'protective process'. |
| Hidden feelings | Emotions that are out of conscious awareness which drive our behaviours. |
| Insight | The process of persons becoming more aware of what they were previously unaware of. |
| Interpretations | One of the main tools of psychodynamic therapy, the therapist's way of helping the person to understand, or gain insight into what is going on, in order to bring their unconscious feelings into conscious awareness and make sense of them. |
| Projection | The process whereby 'unwanted' aspects of the self are 'put into' another; in this process the other person is seen as having the unwanted aspects, e.g. the other person is seen as being (but does not really feel) upset by the person who has projected their upset. |
| Transference | The feelings that the person has about the therapist, which are likely to be influenced by the person's experiences of relationships in the past. |
| Unconscious | The process of when something is out of our conscious awareness. |
| Unconscious communications | The ways in which we communicate what we are not aware of, e.g. in our dreams. |

## REFERENCES


Leiper, R. (2006) 'Psychodynamic formulation. A prince betrayed and disinherited'. in L. Johnstone and R. Dallos (eds), *Formulation in Psychology and Psychotherapy: Making Sense of People's Problems*. London: Routledge.

Lemma, A. (2006) *Introduction to the Practice of Psychoanalytic Psychotherapy*. Chichester Wiley.

Lemma, A., Roth, A. D. and Pilling, S. (2010) *The Competences Required to Deliver Effective Psychoanalytic/Psychodynamic Therapy.* Research Department of Clinical, Educational and Health Psychology UCL. Available at: www.ucl.ac.uk/clinical-psychology/CORE/psychodynamic_framework.htm (accessed August 2010).

Malan, D. H. (2007) *Individual Psychotherapy and the Science of Psychodynamics*, (2nd edn). London: Hodder Education.

Molnos, A. (1995) *A Question of Time: Essentials of Brief Dynamic Psychotherapy*. London: Karnac.

## Worksheet 5.1

## Assessment

This table gives us some ideas of what the therapist will look for in the assessment period.

| | Example questions/things to think about | Your thoughts as therapist |
|---|---|---|
| Facts | What brings you to therapy at this point in your life?<br>• How do they explain their difficulties?<br>• Do they acknowledge an emotional element?<br>• Do you notice any themes? | |
| Strategies/ways of coping | How did you cope when X happened?<br>• Be aware of any risk issues in ways of coping, e.g. self-harm.<br>• What are the risks of this person engaging in therapy?<br>• How do they cope with painful or difficult feelings? | |
| Relationships | Tell me about your family?<br>What words would you use to describe your mother/father?<br>How would you describe your childhood? What memories do you have from childhood?<br>Who were you closest to as a child?<br>Who are you closest to now?<br>• Are there any common themes/feelings in the person's descriptions?<br>• Do they have at least one supportive relationship outside of therapy?<br>• Are there some feelings that are notably absent? | |
| Goals/aims | What are your hopes for coming here?<br>What would it mean if your life was different?<br>• Are these goals achievable?<br>• Are the aims in line with what psychodynamic therapy can offer?<br>• Do they believe that change is possible?<br>• What are the consequences of change? | |

## Worksheet 5.2

## Triangle of conflict

The triangle of conflict is the basis of a psychodynamic formulation. It has three components: defences, anxieties, hidden feelings. Here's one for jotting down your own notes.

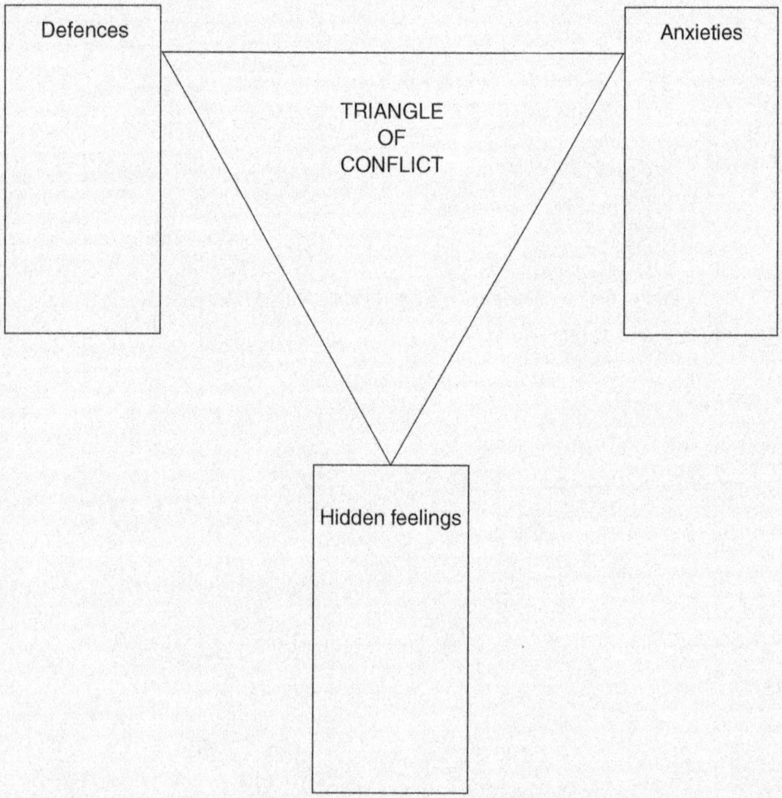

## Worksheet 5.3

## Defences

We all use defence mechanisms to some extent; they are the ways that we deal with distressing and unwanted anxiety and emotions and are often outside our awareness. If defences are used appropriately, and are adaptive, they may never become problematic. There are endless lists of defences, but here are a few examples.

| *Term* | Definition | Example |
|---|---|---|
| ***Repression*** | A distressing thought/ memory is kept out of conscious awareness, to reduce anxiety. | A murderous intent to kill. These thoughts often return through processes such as our dreams. |
| ***Denial*** | Refusing to acknowledge that the source of anxiety exists, we are unaware that we are denying it. | Continuing to make tea for a partner after they have left you, refusing to believe they have gone. |
| ***Regression*** | Reverting back to an earlier state when we are acutely distressed. | When admitted to hospital we become very needy and appear more childlike. |
| ***Projection*** | Putting an unwanted impulse we have onto someone else (not consciously). | An unfaithful wife becomes very jealous of her husband and suspects him of being unfaithful. |
| ***Rationalisation*** | Explaining something rationally. | Justifying failing an exam: 'I didn't fail the exam because I didn't study hard enough, I failed because the exam questions were worded badly.' |

*(Continued)*

*(Continued)*

| *Term* | **Definition** | **Example** |
|---|---|---|
| *Intellectualisation* | Changing our feelings into thoughts and focusing on thoughts rather than dealing with emotions. | When a loved one is diagnosed with dementia, we may look up every fact on dementia to avoid dealing with our sadness and feelings about the diagnosis. |
| *Displacement* | Moving an impulse from one person/object to another. | You are angry with a work colleague so you go home and yell at your partner. |
| *Sublimation* | Transform an impulse into something helpful or desirable. | An angry person takes up boxing or digs the garden. |
| *Acting out* | Behaving in a way that symbolises what we are unable/unwilling to express. | Having a temper tantrum rather than talking through how we feel. |
| *Reaction formation* | When we do or think the opposite to what we are feeling. | When you are angry with someone and so you make an extra effort to be nice to them. |
| *Somatisation* | Converting feelings into physical symptoms. | A relationship ends and rather than feel upset our feelings become expressed as stomach ache/sickness. |

## Worksheet 5.4

## Transference

Recognising and understanding transference patterns can be really challenging. The following tips give you ideas of what to look out for, and possible responses.

| Transference pattern | Signs from person | Therapist's feelings (countertransference) | What you might do |
|---|---|---|---|
| Idealised therapist | • Excessive compliments.<br>• Agreeing with everything therapist says.<br>• Wearing similar clothes to therapist. | Competence: 'I'm doing a great job.'<br>Satisfaction: 'I'm good at my job.'<br>Confusion: 'I'm unsure what the person really thinks.'<br>Frustration: 'I don't know what to do about this.' | Explore the person's expectations of therapy and what they find helpful.<br>Explore person's sense of self and self-belief.<br>Trace back to roots and relationships that have also evoked these feelings. |
| Therapist as expert | • Ascribes power and authority to therapist.<br>• Looks for answers, solutions and advice.<br>• Waits for therapist to impose structure or ask questions. | Expertness: 'I'm great at this, I know all the answers.'<br>Anxiety:'I don't have all the answers.'<br>Self-doubt: 'I don't know what I'm doing.'<br>Feeling incompetent: 'I can't help this person.' | Explore the person's need for advice and lack of confidence in own ability.<br>Try to help the person trace this back to their roots, i.e. who has made them feel that they can't make decisions. |

*(Continued)*

*(Continued)*

| **Transference pattern** | **Signs from person** | **Therapist's feelings (countertransference)** | **What you might do** |
|---|---|---|---|
| Therapist as a threat | • Defensive and guarded in response to therapist.<br>• Suspicious, distrustful.<br>• Engaging and withdrawing during the course of a session. | Uneasy, uncomfortable. Unsure of when to question and be silent. Withdrawal from person. Concern about doing damage to person.<br>Hopelessness: 'I can't work with this person'.<br>Feeling dislike for the person.<br>The feeling of dread before seeing the person. | Focus on issues of trust. Can they name their concerns about you/the therapy? Can they explore what this might be about (now and past)?<br>Be explicit and open with the person and involve them in the decision making about therapy.<br>Explore the impact of trust on therapy. |
| Therapist as rescuer | • Neediness, demanding and helplessness.<br>• View of self as victim. | Urge to rescue and nurture the person. Treading carefully and fearful of making interpretations.<br>Fear of pushing the person too far.<br>Engagement in a lengthy therapy contract. | Explore experiences that may have contributed to helplessness (now and past).<br>Explore relationships that may have been over-supportive. |

# 6 SYSTEMIC THERAPIES

Amie Smith and
Stephen Weatherhead

Systemic therapy is a way of thinking as much as it is a therapy. It can be applied in many different settings and in many different ways. Its primary application in the therapeutic domain is with families, referred to as 'family therapy'. Systemic therapists work collaboratively with the system/family, using techniques such as developing genograms, asking particular types of questions, and sharing reflections with the family on what they have observed and heard during therapy sessions. When combined, these techniques help families to develop new patterns of interaction to overcome previous problems.

## THE MODEL

Systems theory cuts across many different disciplines such as biology, sociology and economics. We are concerned with the system in the context of therapy. In this case, the system is a group of people who are connected in some way. It may be that they work for the same organisation, live in the same care home, or are a family. The family is the most common system in which models of systemic therapy are applied, which is one of the reasons that the terms systemic therapy and family therapy are often used interchangeably. We have opted to refer to the model as 'systemic therapy' because it can be used in so many other systems. Similarly, when we use the term 'family', this can be taken to mean any system.

Systemic therapy emerged from a shift in thinking in the 1950s. At this time therapies were dominated by individual (intra-psychic) thinking that viewed symptoms and problems as existing within the person. Families were viewed as the sum of each individual's psyche. There was a need for therapy that could meet the demands of therapy with families, and out of this need grew systemic therapy. Systemic theory originates from studies in biology that explains patterns within organisms. When applied to humans, systemic theory views an individual's experiences as interpersonal, rather than individual.

Many people new to systemic therapy may assume that you cannot practice it unless you are in a session working with a whole family, and have a team of other professionals working alongside you who offer reflections (i.e. their thoughts about what is going on for the family and in the session). On the contrary, there are many ways of practising systemic therapy that may not look like the traditional family therapy session. Systemic therapy can take place with individuals, couples, families, professional teams, and the therapist may be working alone or as part of a team.

The common factor in each of the forms systemic therapy takes is that they are based on systemic thinking. Systemic thinking is the idea that individuals exist and develop in relationships. Rather than viewing the individual as having a problem within them personally, systemic thinking takes the view that human experiences are best understood and explained in relational terms. In other words, the meaning, maintenance and solutions to a person's distress are connected to their relationships and experiences with other people. Therefore, systemic therapists are interested in the problems that the whole family bring to therapy.

When reading about systemic/family therapy, you will often come across references to 'schools' of family therapy. This refers to the different models that have evolved from the same philosophical foundations. For an overview of the development of systemic therapy, have a read of the section at the end of this chapter.

Many systemic therapists would not feel it is necessary to know the 'cause' of the problem. Instead, they will see the therapist's function as being to:

- Make connections between different levels of relationships (e.g. family, societal, group and cultural).
- Explore the relationship between these levels over time, and make connections between past, present and future.

To fulfil this function, systemic therapists believe that the therapist needs to be open-minded and curious when working with the family. This means that therapists are required to think through their own assumptions and agendas to allow them to be most focused on what is helpful for the family.

In brief, if you are exploring patterns, relationships and connections in therapy, and taking a curious stance to this, then you are likely to be working systemically.

During the therapy session itself, systemic therapists are interested in both the content and process of working with people. This simply means that we are interested in observing how people interact and the ways they tell their stories, as well as giving consideration to what is actually said. Therapists will be looking at non-verbal as well as verbal behaviour to help deepen understandings.

Systemic therapy can at times be relatively short-term. One session can sometimes be enough to identify unhelpful ways of acting and reacting together and result in positive changes. The approach can be useful across the lifespan (Marriot, 2000), but the interactions that occur during systemic therapy may be difficult or stressful for some people to understand. This is one reason why it can sometimes be useful to have individual therapy available as well.

> Although this chapter will focus on systemic approaches to direct working, the systemic approach also offers a helpful framework when undertaking indirect work, such as consultation, training, and networking. For more information on applying systemic ideas indirectly, see Harper and Spellman (1994).

In summary, systemic therapy is a model that can be used with families, couples, colleagues or any group in some form of relationship. The approach aims to explore the connections and interactions between those relationships. It is concerned with what is happening during therapy, as well as what is being said. It has no specific time-schedule, setting, age-group, or type of problem within which it should or should not be applied.

## APPLICATION

Like many other therapies, there is no set way of doing systemic therapy and it does not follow a set sequence. However, there are number of techniques and strategies that can be used in systemic therapy. Some of the key techniques are covered here and are grouped under the core elements of a systemic approach. There are of course many techniques to consider, but the ones we have chosen to focus on are: contexts and using genograms; circular thinking and questioning; observations and reflections; hypothesising and formulating.

> Systemic therapists believe that the important work occurs outside the therapy room. Therefore, the start of sessions may focus on what family members have noticed happening between sessions.

### Contexts and using genograms

Systemic therapists pay attention to the family or the system's background, what is going on around them, and how they are organised. Systemic theorists also believe that the family is an open system, which means that they are open to and influenced by other factors, such as the wider society, culture, the economy and other influences. They also believe that the family changes over time and problems may arise due to difficulties in adapting to these changes. For example, children going to school may lead to anxiety about being separated from caregivers.

One of the most useful ways of summarising this information is to draw a genogram. Genograms (a.k.a. family trees or maps) are a tool to help therapists summarise and gather extensive amounts of information about family members, histories and relationships between people. They are accessible and allow themes to be drawn out. This is important because those themes may recur across generations and relate to underpinning beliefs. Obviously it isn't possible to include all information on a genogram; they should develop during the course of therapy, and include snippets of pertinent information at any given time.

> **Example:** Mark and Lisa were referred because of conflict around their parenting roles. Lisa wanted to re-establish her career after childbirth. Drawing a genogram generated a discussion that revealed a strong belief in Mark's family that women should be the main caregivers. This was in contrast to the beliefs and views on Lisa's side of the family. Lisa, her mother and her sister all had strong career ambitions and believed in equality of genders with regard to parenting roles. Drawing the genogram (Figure 6.1) allowed the couple to develop a greater understanding of what was contributing to their beliefs and influencing the current situation.

Creating a genogram with a family early in therapy can help to engage several family members on a task. This relies on the therapist being active in asking questions in relation to the genogram. For example, genograms may be useful in:

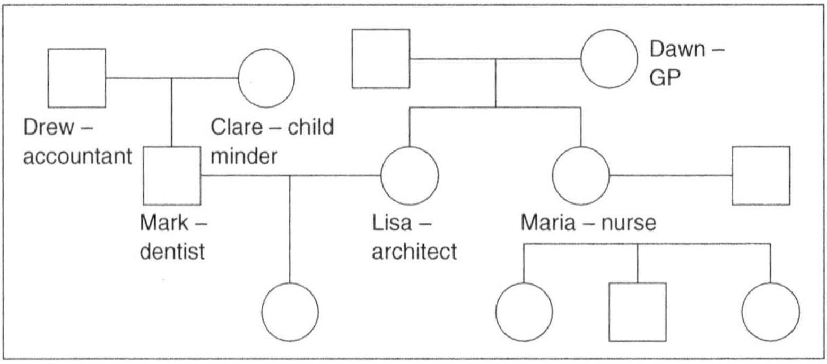


**Figure 6.1** Mark and Lisa's genogram

- Finding out about important events (such as bereavements and family members leaving home) and how people have adapted to these. Often it can be useful for the therapist to draw a time-line of important events alongside the genogram to help organise this information.

> There are lots of different symbols and keys you can use when drawing genograms. For some examples, see Gerson and Petry (2008).

- Finding out what are the ideas and beliefs that people in the family share or who does not share these beliefs.
- Finding out what rules exist in the family, what routines they have or who has what role (e.g. the men always take the bins out on bin day, the women always cook tea).
- Helping families and therapists to consider relationships and patterns of interaction from different people's perspectives. For Mark and Lisa in the example above, developing the genogram helped Mark to understand why his mother-in-law had been so supportive of Lisa going back to work.
- Allowing the therapist to observe patterns of interaction as they happen in the session. Some things to observe include:
    - Who in the family takes the lead.
    - Who speaks the most/least.
    - Who agrees/disagrees.
    - Whose views are ignored.
    - How the family reaches agreements.

## Circular thinking and questioning

Linear thinking/questions are direct, and often focus on cause and effect (e.g. X leads to Y or she is depressed because her cat died) and can be very useful in gathering information, particularly in the early stages of therapy. For example one may ask 'How long have you been married?', 'How many children do you have?', 'What do you do if you are angry?', 'What do you do after that?'.

Linear theorists will be looking for the root of the problem; what causes it, how did it start (see Figure 6.2). However, systemic theorists work on the premise that humans are more complex than a cause-and-effect model would suggest, because of their interactions with others. So, systemic theorists believe that our understanding of something is limited if we just see it on its own (i.e. think linearly).

Our understanding is enhanced if we see the 'thing' in relation to something else. This involves thinking about how things are connected, how they feed back into each other and the differences between things. This way of thinking of things as interconnected is called 'circular thinking'. In circular explanations

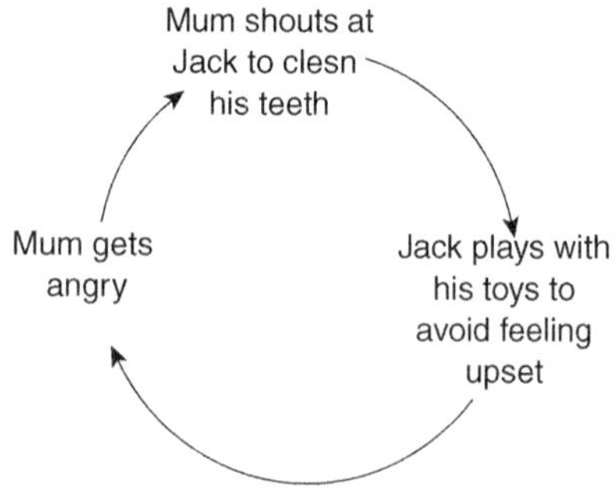
Mum shouts at Jack to clesn his teeth
Jack plays with his toys to avoid feeling upset
Mum gets angry

**Figure 6.2** Linear theory

each person's behaviours, beliefs or feelings are explained and maintained by the other person's actions, beliefs or feelings; things happen in a circular pattern.

Because things happen in a circular fashion in systemic therapy, it is not helpful to look for one cause of a problem, who started it or who is to blame. Finding a cause is often impossible, like asking 'Which came first, the chicken or the egg?'. Rather, systemic therapists would look to find out about the repetitive patterns that have become a habit for the family (or system). Thinking circularly enables therapists to gain information and form ideas about the complex family relationships, patterns and interactions, that is, how family members relate to each other, how members' beliefs, actions and feelings affect them and other members, how the whole family rules affect each member. Therapists would try to work out how these patterns are developing, how they are being influenced by the family, and how the patterns are influencing all the members of the family. One way to find these things out is by using circular questions. For example, 'What does Jim feel about your worries about your body?', 'How did you develop the view that you are a bad person?', 'Why does your mum think you get sad?', 'Who do you think finds things hardest since your Nan passed away?'

> If you're feeling particularly brave and want to read a good examination of the philosophy and practice of circular questioning, try Karl Tomm or Gregory Batesen's writing on the topic.

Circular questions aim to make the family aware of new information (e.g. new patterns that they may not have been aware of before therapy). This allows them to take a step back and observe themselves and the problem from a different perspective. In turn, this may open up new possibilities for the family. Circular questions also help to add more information by drawing out connections and looking into differences in a non-confrontational manner (because the focus is not on one person or event as no one thing is to 'blame'). The differences may relate to behaviours, feelings, beliefs, relationships, or any of them in combination. The hope is that highlighting differences and taking a different perspective may help to change some of the unhelpful circular patterns.

**Example:** Tammy (13 years old), her sister Stacey (19 years old), mother Bridget and father Mick were attending a family session following concerns about Tammy self-harming. It became apparent that Tammy and Mick dealt with their feelings by 'bottling them up', whereas Stacey and Bridget frequently dealt with emotions by getting angry. A series of circular questions helped explore how the family processed and communicated feelings, for example: 'Stacey, what would Tammy say about how you deal with difficult feelings?', 'How does not talking calmly about feelings affect relationships in the family?', 'Bridget, what would happen if Mick spoke more about his feelings?', 'Mick, why do you think Bridget feels so angry about the family difficulties?', 'Tammy, what would happen if you got angry in the way you have described other family members as doing?'

One final note on circular questions; they are a quite difficult idea to grasp (even for us as therapists). Using puppets, drawing and play can help to describe the concept to younger people. However, it is important to remember that young children and people with cognitive difficulties may find it particularly difficult to take another person's point of view.

## Observations and reflections

In systemic approaches the therapists take a position of 'observing', which involves them taking a neutral stance, stepping back and looking at what is happening in the system. This approach makes it easier to select, organise and highlight the sequences of behaviour and interactions between the family members.

There is always more than one perspective, and no definitive 'right'. Different observers may describe the same family differently and come up with different ideas. All ideas are important in therapy and can give valuable information that may help the family to move forward. Each observer's idea may be shared with the family. This could be a way to highlight both helpful and unhelpful patterns. Again the hope is that speaking about those patterns can enable people to develop the helpful ones, and limit the unhelpful ones.

**Example:** During a family session the youngest child (Melissa, 6 years old) didn't speak and no-one else asked her point of view. Observers shared with the family that they had noticed this and wondered how this left Melissa feeling? As a result of this question, Melissa was given the opportunity to speak and said that she didn't feel like anyone wanted to hear her opinion, because no one ever asked her, and this made her feel like she wasn't important. The session progressed by allowing Melissa and her family to explore alternative things people did or said that helped make her feel more important.

Systemic therapists believe that the therapy system itself (i.e. the therapist(s) and family members in the session) has its own dynamics and beliefs. For example, at the first session the whole system may hold hope of change or, on the contrary, feel a sense of hopelessness that things will never change.

This means that therapists and observers need to be reflective and open to how their own views and experiences may be influencing their behaviour and thinking in the session. For example, thinking about how the therapist's own family experiences, or how their current life events, may influence how they see the family and family member's actions is crucial. In the above example, the therapist may have experienced a similar situation to Melissa when he felt unheard, and this may influence how he relates to Melissa in the session, either consciously asking her more questions or, similar to her family members, he may not include her in conversations. Either way, it is important that the therapist acknowledges his own feelings and beliefs in order to be able to remain neutral/impartial and curious.

> We can all be guilty of making negative comments, or being involved in unhelpful dynamics. Sharing observations and reflections with families helps keep this in check.

Systemic therapists may also take breaks mid-way or at the end of the session in order to have time and space to reflect. This is viewed as an important way of gaining more understanding of the family. The therapist may spend time at the end of the session making reflective notes. These notes are not about the content of the session but are focused on things like:

- What stood out for me during the session?
- How did I feel during the session?
- What else am I curious about?

## Hypothesising and formulating

Systemic therapists believe that the ideas (hypotheses) professionals may form about a family based on the information they have are changeable over time and in different situations. Therefore, these ideas need to be revised as we learn more about the family. Therapists will test ideas out by discussing them with the family, often using statements such as 'I wonder if …', 'I am curious whether ...' to hear the family members' views.

Very often in systemic therapy sessions you will hear the therapist check their understanding with the family in a short statement, for example, 'Let me just check that I have understood this: you feel that if you made your mum a cup of tea, then your mum would know that you appreciated her? Have I understood that correctly?' These statements are used to:

- Help the therapist to organise the information they have heard.
- Let the family know they have heard what has been said, correctly.
- Allow the therapist to follow the statement with a question that will develop further understanding, for example, 'What would your mum say or do that would tell you that she knows you appreciate her?'

Systemic therapists will also take note of the emotions and behaviour (verbal and non-verbal) that are happening in the session and use this to form ideas. For example, they may ask: 'Sarah is looking upset, what do you think is so upsetting for her when we are discussing your relationship?', 'I noticed your face changed as your mum started to discuss anger, I wonder whether anger is around for you in today's session?'

> Vetere and Dallos (2003) go into more depth about systemic formulation and how other approaches can be integrated into the systemic framework.

All these ideas will be used to gain a shared understanding and description (a formulation) of the family relationships, and of the problem. It is important that systemic therapists work with the family in collaboration to reach a shared formulation, rather than the therapist being an expert putting a formulation onto the family. Spending time to build up trust and making sure every member of the system feels able to have a voice and be listened to can be a difficult task. However, the systemic therapist needs to encourage people to share differences in opinions.

By sharing formulations and ideas, systemic therapists can help families and systems to gain a greater insight into their situation, which can help to:

- Improve the communication within the family.
- Make members become aware of behaviours that are acted out unconsciously.
- Lead members to change or reduce these behaviours.

Systemic therapists believe that the family hold the expertise in finding the solution to their difficulties. In sessions, therapists will ask about the things the family have done to try to solve the problems and what has worked. If therapy progresses over several sessions, therapists will be looking for examples of solutions and successes that have occurred between each session. The therapist may for example, ask 'What have you noticed that has been different since we last met?'

When successes (however small) have been highlighted, the therapist will then spend time exploring these successes asking questions (often circular) such as: 'What gave you the idea to do this?', 'So you were able to show your daughter you were pleased by smiling at her, how do you think your smile made her feel?', 'How did she respond?', 'If your mother was here what would she think of that?', 'What gave you the confidence to keep doing this new idea?'

The hope is that by making the family more aware of the details of solutions and successes, and other people's views of these, they can begin to do more of what is working. Over the course of systemic therapy, whether it is one session or ten, the hope is that the family will be able to focus on changes that have occurred. The conversations will be more about the solutions that the family are working on rather than the difficulties. The overall aim is to enable the individuals and the family as a whole to continue to find solutions and maintain change, once therapy has ended.

Narrative therapy and solution-focused therapy use a lot of the same techniques as systemic therapy, e.g. externalising. This is because they are all built on similar philosophies.

Finally, at the end of therapy, systemic therapists may offer the family time to review the process of therapy. This can be useful to help prevent future difficulties and enable the family to feel that they have the skills and resources to cope with future problems. In the review the therapist may ask questions such as: 'What has been most useful/least useful for the family through therapy?', 'What has been gained/lost for the family through therapy?', 'What would the family do differently if, in the future, difficulties occurred?'

Within this chapter we have tried to give an overview of what we see as the core components of systemic therapy. These include: contexts and using genograms; circular thinking and questioning; observations and reflections; hypothesising and formulating. A purist from any single school may give a slightly different slant, or choose alternative areas to focus on. However, hopefully this chapter has introduced you to what we feel are the foundations of systemic therapies. As with any therapy, if you find this model sits well with you, we would strongly encourage you to explore some of the more specialised texts that are available.

## CASE STUDY

The Abdullah family were referred to family therapy by their general practitioner 18 months after their daughter (Dina) was diagnosed with Lupus. The whole family were struggling with life since the diagnosis, and wanted help with managing the problem. Developing the genogram in Figure 6.3 helped identify some of the factors that had made it so difficult to manage the diagnosis.

Whilst drawing the genogram, the therapist was curious about how Abdi and Sara met. Through this conversation the therapist drew a time-line and learned about the family history, their stories and each family member's beliefs and values. Abdi and his family were brought up living a religious life in Saudi Arabia. After Mo's death, Abdi and his mother Lila moved to the UK to allow Abdi to pursue his career. Abdi married Sara shortly after settling in the UK. They bought a home, which had a 'granny flat' for Lila. Sara's parents (Peter and Anne) had showed dismay at their daughter's marriage. Abdi had never felt welcomed by them. According to

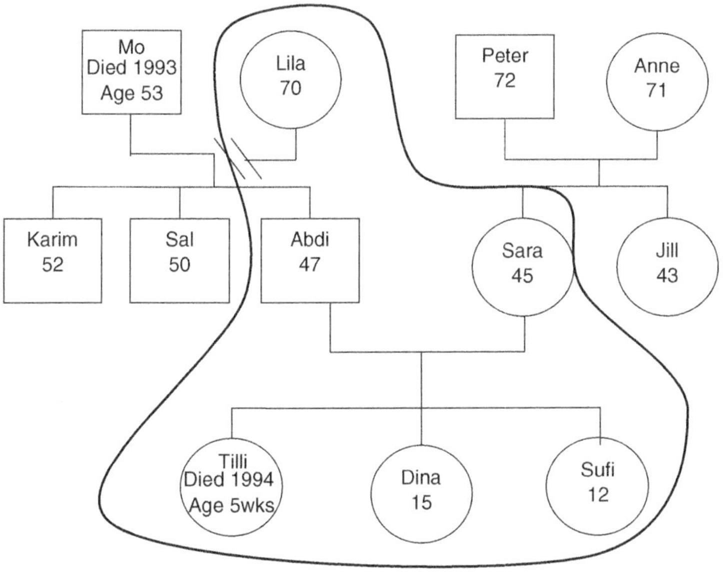


**Figure 6.3** Genogram for the Abdullah family

*(Continued)*

*(Continued)*

Sara, her parents were 'awkward' about discussing her and Abdi's relationship and her father had declined to give a speech at the wedding. Sara described her father as 'a bit racist' and had told her that their marriage 'could never work'.

When Sara soon became pregnant, Abdi, Sara and Lila were very pleased; however Sara's parents were not as joyful. Unfortunately the pregnancy had a number of complications, the baby (Tilli) was born very prematurely and died aged five weeks. Sara experienced what she described as 'a dark time' after Tilli died. She feared that there was something wrong with her, despite having no medical problems prior to the pregnancy. Whilst discussing this during the session Sara also said, for the first time, that part of her was worried that her father may have been 'right' about them (Abdi and Sara), and that their relationship couldn't work. A part of her was concerned that the loss of their baby was somehow connected to their ethnic differences:

*Sara*: I don't know about this stuff, genetics and that, but maybe this has all happened because we're not s'posed to mix so much.

*Therapist*: What do you think Abdi's view is on that?

*Sara*: We've never talked about it, but I reckon he'd think it was daft. He knows about science, and I know he loves me.

*Therapist*: You know he loves you?

*Sara*: Yeah, he loves me, and he said what happened to little Tilli and what's happened to Dina is horrible bad luck. I guess I know really that we do work, and that it's nothing to do with us being from different backgrounds. It's just a worry.

*Therapist*: Listening to what you're saying makes me wonder who this is a worry for?

*Sara*: It's my dad's really; I reckon his views are wrong about this.

Following this, the reflecting team who were sat in another corner of the room had an opportunity to speak. They commented on a number of things including:

- how much strength the family have shown in working through the challenges they have faced;
- how interesting it was that Sara used the words 'my dad's views about this', rather than labelling it as her own views.

*(Continued)*

It was this second comment that seemed to strike a chord with the whole family. It was Sufi who reflected on it first:

*Sufi*: It's right you know, all the things that go bad, granddad blames on us being mixed race. I love him, but he's got weird views sometimes. I think that's why we can't talk about this stuff much.

*Sara*: What stuff?

*Sufi*: You know the illness, Tilli, I know it worries dad.

*Abdi*: You are a wise person, Sufi. I don't like talking about it because a part of me is scared he's right. My dad used to say everything was down to God, and I didn't believe that. So, I put everything down to science. Then things like this happen, which neither religion nor science can explain, and I don't know what to think. I'm scared.

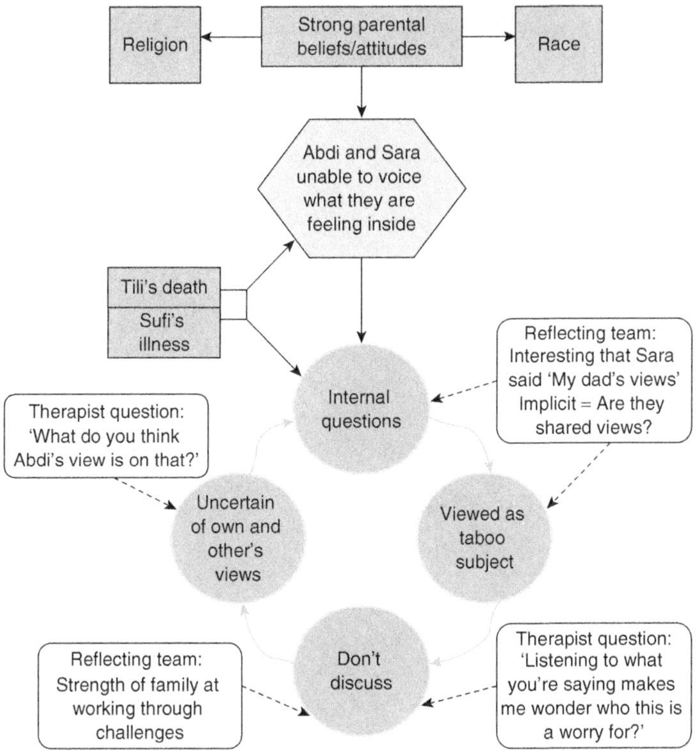


**Figure 6.4** The Abdullah family's therapy pattern in progress

*(Continued)*

*(Continued)*

The family went on to say that this was the first time Abdi had ever admitted being scared. This opened many discussions about how they were all scared. Sara and Abdi were scared because they couldn't find an explanation and the future was unpredictable, and the children were scared because they could see that it scared their parents. It felt at the time that this was a significant shift for the family. There was further evidence of this at the following session, when the reflecting team noted that the family sat closer to each other, Abdi held Sufi's hand a couple of times, and they shared a joke at one point (the first time this had happened during a session).

This is just an excerpt from the process and content of five sessions with the family. However, it highlights that exploring all the family members' views, reflecting observations back and picking up on the nuances in conversations, helped to change the circular pattern that had caused the family to avoid talking about certain aspects of their problem. Changing this pattern introduced a psychological and visible shift, increasing the family's strength to deal with their difficulties (see Figure 6.4).

## THE DEVELOPMENT OF SYSTEMIC THERAPIES

Many theorists have looked back over the decades during which systemic therapies have developed, and have generally drawn out three specific stages (or orders) to its development, which coincide with the developments in the wider field of psychology. If any of what follows inspires you to read on, Dallos and Draper (2005) provide more detailed information about the three phases and the cultural landscapes that influenced each phase.

The first stage began in the 1960s. In this stage the family was viewed as a system and the therapist was seen as outside of the system. Problems were viewed as serving a function within the family, for example a child's difficult behaviour served the function of taking attention away from parents arguing. Therapists focused on the behavioural sequences and patterns of the family and looked at how the problem may be serving the function of maintaining the stability of the family system. These views were similar to the behavioural or psychodynamic views, which dominated the field of psychology at this time. In this stage the therapist was seen as 'acting on' the family; as an expert they could exert change upon the family during therapy.

The second stage, which began in the 1980s, viewed the therapist as part of the system, moving away from the idea of the therapist as an expert.

Within the wider field of psychology, cognitive theories started to dominate, with a focus on cognitions, meanings and beliefs. This influenced systemic thinking, and within this stage there was a focus on each individual within the system (including the therapist) having their own personal, unique view and expectations of the world and of the family and its members. The aim of the therapist was to work alongside the family to co-create new and more useful ways of the family viewing the situation.

The 1960s–80s saw the emergence of different schools of family therapy: structural family therapy (the founder was Salvador Minuchin), strategic family therapy (a big name from this school is Jay Hayley) and systemic/Milan family therapy (big names from this group include Luigi Boscolo, Gianfranco Cecchin, Mara Selvini Palazzoli). Each of these schools applied the principles of systems theory to family therapy, but they focused on and applied the principles slightly differently. For example, the goal of structural therapy is to change the family structure, the goal of strategic is to change the pattern of interaction in the family, and the goal of systemic/Milan therapy is to change the family beliefs and rules. It is a big task to provide an overview of all the schools of family therapy, beyond the scope of this chapter, and we have chosen to mention only three here. If you are interested in reading a more detailed introduction to these three schools, see Hayes (1991).

The move into the third stage was influenced by the development of social constructionism and focuses on how contexts, particularly language and culture, shape the expectations and actions of family members. Out of social constructionism grew therapies such as narrative and solution-focused approaches, and hence systemic therapies share many things in common with these approaches. In this stage more emphasis is placed on how wider socially formed ideas and assumptions, related to gender, race or class (that are embedded and communicated in language), shape the family. The therapist's role in this stage focuses on bringing these ideas into the awareness of the family, with the view that being more aware of these can help the family to be less trapped by them.

## GLOSSARY

| | |
|---|---|
| Content | What is actually said during therapy sessions. |
| Contexts | Situations in which the family systems operate and may include amongst other things, family networks, wider society, culture, the economy. |
| Circular questions | Questions aimed at encouraging the consideration of an issue, from a different perspective. Often focused on the interactions between different aspects of the issue at hand. |
| Formulation | A shared understanding of a situation, problem or possible solutions. Often accompanied by a diagram showing interactions. |

| | |
|---|---|
| Genogram | A family tree, which may contain other information such as cultural beliefs, ages, jobs. |
| Hypothesis | A tentative theory on any feature or thing, such as the problem, relationships, things that are happening inside and outside therapy. |
| Process | What is observed to be happening during a therapy session, for example body language, changes in mood and hesitations. |
| Reflections | These are simply thoughts about what has been said, heard and witnessed. |
| Reflecting team | This is a group of observers whose task is to observe what is happening in the therapy, verbal and non-verbal communication. The observers will then think about what they have witnessed and offer their reflections to the therapist, and the family. |
| System | A group of people with a shared connection, the most common of which is a family. |

## REFERENCES

Carr, A. (2006) *Family Therapy: Concepts, Process and Practice.* Chilchester: Wiley-Blackwell.
Dallos, R. and Draper, R. (2005) *An Introduction to Family Therapy, Systemic Theory and Practice.* Maidenhead: Open University Press.
Gerson, R. and Petry, S. (2008) *Genograms: Assessment and Intervention.* London: Norton.
Harper, D. and Spellman, D. (1994) 'Consultation to a professional network: Reflections of a would-be consultant', *Journal of Family Therapy, 16,* 389-399.
Hayes, H. (1991) 'A re-introduction to family therapy clarification of three schools', *Australian and New Zealand Journal of Family Therapy, 12* (1), 27-43.
Marriot, A. (2000) *Family Therapy with Older Adults and their Families.* Oxford: Winslow.
Vetere, A. and Dallos, R. (2003) *Working Systemically with Families: Formulation, Intervention and Evaluation.* London: Karnac.

# Worksheet 6.1

## Genograms

Genograms are family trees, with a bit more about them. They can include a whole range of information from ages to cultural beliefs. They are an evolving document, which can be used in different parts of therapy, and are often accompanied by a time-line of significant events. Useful texts showing genograms and the associated symbols include Gerson and Petry (2008) and Carr (2006).

### Where do I start?

- Start with those involved in therapy, then work backwards through generations.
- Children are placed in birth order from left to right.
- In couples, the male goes on the left and female on the right.
- Males are represented by a square and females by a circle.
- Draw a circle around all the people who live in the same house.

### How much detail do I include?

- As much as the family want to. They may want to include pets, friends and so on.
- Always ask if there is anything else to include.
- Use a large piece of paper to allow more information to be added later.
- Organisation of complicated genograms can be aided by using different colours and having a key somewhere on the page.

### Who will see the genogram?

- This should be discussed with the family, but it can be useful to include information other professionals may find useful. For example:

    - medics may wish to know about the family history of conditions such as dementia or heart disease (perhaps represent by shading the symbol in a different colour);
    - social services may be interested in risk-related issues (maybe note on a time-line), or the closeness of relationships. Often a double line between two symbols shows a close relationship, and a zigzag denotes a conflictual relationship.

### What about potentially sensitive stuff?

- Introducing any sensitive issues is a delicate subject. It may feel less challenging to note things such as prison sentences or violence on the time-line.
- Some points such as religion, sexuality or group membership may be shown by using different colours to shade symbols.
- There are a few different ways in which a death may be noted, such as drawing an X through the symbol that contains years of birth and death, drawing a Christian cross or writing RIP inside the symbol, or simply putting deceased along with relevant dates and age.
- Include whatever the family want to include; do not be pushy, but do enquire gently.

## Worksheet 6.2

## Circular questions

Many different theorists have categorised circular questions differently and called the categories by different names. In the table below we give just a few examples of questions, but rather than re-name and re-categorise these (again!) we have grouped them by aims of how you could use them in therapy.

| Circular question | Examples |
|---|---|
| To enquire about what other people do, feel and believe in interactions. | • What does your mum do or say that makes you think she thinks you're silly?<br>• When your son says that he hates you, what does your partner do?<br>• What do you think your partner feels when he hears your son say this?<br>• What ideas do you think your partner may have about that? |
| To enquire about how people differ in the way they respond to situations or how the problem is different and changes over time. | • Who is the most/least worried about the problem?<br>• On a scale of 0–10, how alone do you think your son feels when his sister tells him to 'get over it'?<br>• On a scale of 0–10, how bad has arguing been this week? |
| To enquire into changes in people's behaviour which helped change relationships before and after a specific event. | • Did you see your son's relationship with your daughter improve before or after he changed schools? |
| To enquire about the future and differences in opinion with regards to imagined situations in the past, current or future. | • How might the problem change in the future?<br>• What do you think your mum would think about the way you are behaving in five years' time? |
| To offer alternative perspectives. | • What do you think grandma thinks of your behaviour at home?<br>• If I asked your friend, what do you think they would say about your behaviour? |

## Worksheet 6.3

## Reflecting teams

One of the ways in which the principles of observation and reflection are used in family therapy is by using a reflecting team. This is a team of therapists whose role is to observe the family system and share their reflections with the family. There are many different ways this can take place. Perhaps the most traditional is to observe through a one-way mirror, but other examples include:

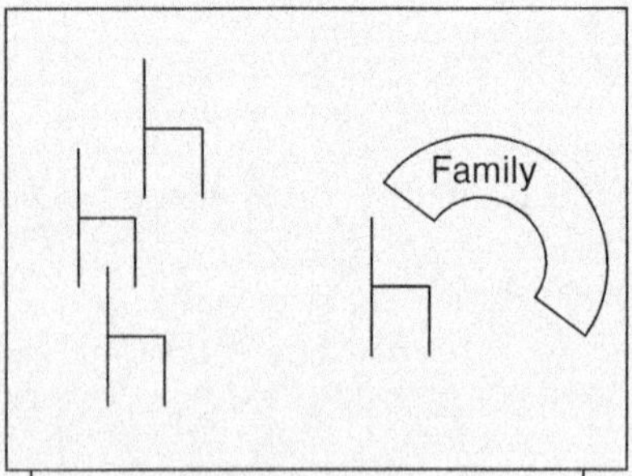

The team sitting in a group, away from the family but in the same room.

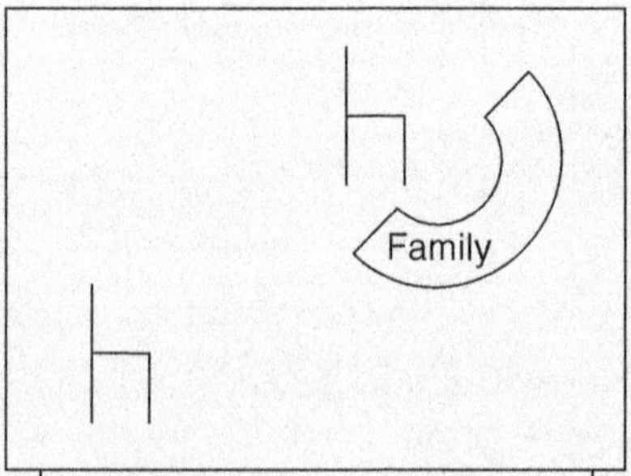

Another therapist, sitting in a group, away from the family but in the same room.

The reflecting team observes the therapy session and, at agreed times, has a conversation with the main therapist about the session. Examples of how to do this include:

- Swapping places, to have a discussion in their team in front of the family.
- Going into a room away from the family, discussing their observations with the therapist. The therapist can then feed back to the family.

The observing team may also help the therapist in the session by giving ideas and feedback via an ear-piece, or a telephone in the room.

Regardless of method, common questions that the observing team will be asking themselves are:

- What stood out for me?
- What questions did this raise for me?
- What would I like to understand more fully?
- How did listening to this impact on me?

# Worksheet 6.4

## Reflections

Here are a number of factors to keep in mind and watch out for when structuring reflections during systemic family therapy.

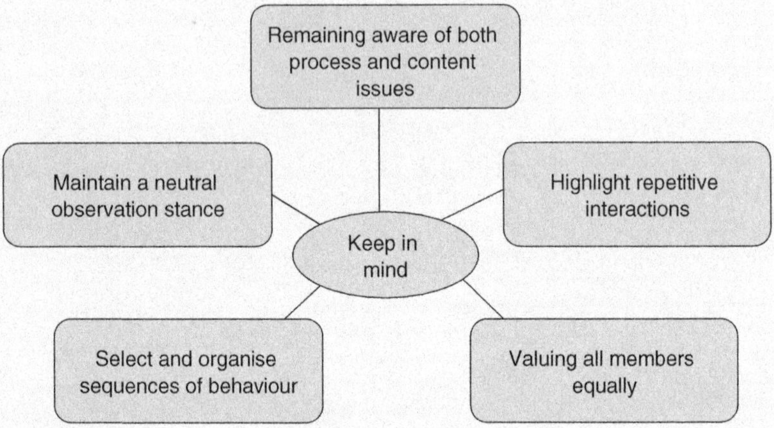


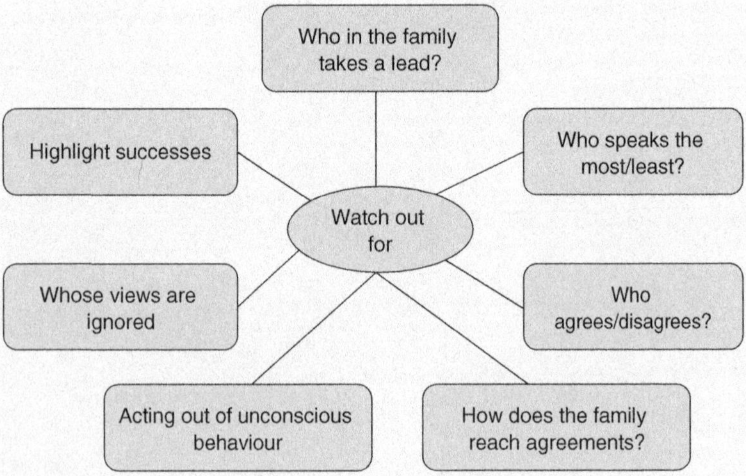


**Process**: What is observed to be happening during a therapy session; for example, body language, changes in mood and hesitations.

**Content**: What is actually said during therapy sessions.

# 7 NARRATIVE THERAPY

Stephen Weatherhead

Narrative therapy is one of the more recently developed therapeutic models, and is very much continuing to evolve. It is built on a poststructuralist philosophy, which views knowledge, power and the stories people live by as inseparable. The therapy aims to explore and re-shape problematic stories, using techniques such as externalisation, deconstruction and the identification of unique outcomes. Narrative therapeutic practice often incorporates indirect forms of therapy, such as the use of therapeutic documents and celebrations involving others, all of which are intended to reinforce the gains made during therapy.

## THE MODEL

The defining principle of narrative therapy is that our identity is built on a series of stories, some of which are privileged whilst others are suppressed. Narrative therapy looks to unpick (deconstruct) and evaluate what has led to problematic stories dominating a person's life. By considering the usefulness and restrictiveness of these stories, as well as searching for exceptions to the rule, richer (thickened) narratives can be developed.

Of the primary models available to therapists, narrative therapy has its philosophical roots most visible. However, it is not necessary to be a master of philosophy to be a good narrative therapist; even the purist accepts skipping out of the more challenging aspects if they are off-putting. Still, it could be argued that the more we understand the roots of the model, the more proficiently we can apply it.

> If you do want to read a bit more about the poststructuralist philosophy that provides the backdrop to narrative therapy, an overview is provided at the end of this chapter.

For now, just keep in mind three issues that cross directly from philosophy into narrative therapy as a model for practice: knowledge, power and language.

They are interlinked and provide the backdrop and core of people's narratives, as well as the tools for therapeutic interventions.

- *Knowledge* – Dominant knowledge serves to reduce the autonomy of a person and cause problematic narratives to feel permanent. Unpicking (deconstructing) this assumed knowledge, and valuing previously marginalised (subjugated) knowledge, allows for alternative stories to emerge.
- *Power* – Modern power is a form of social control that limits identity (White, 2007: 268). The result is thin descriptions, void of contexts such as race, class, gender, sexuality, and the many other discourses that have been utilised as a means of oppression throughout history.
- *Language* – 'We constitute our lives and relationships through language' (White and Epston, 1990: 27). Therapy from a narrative perspective focuses greatly on the language used to define problems, present alternative stories and search for hidden meanings.

This may seem a little overwhelming, and the thought of applying it to practice even more so, but don't worry as help is at hand. In the next section we outline some specific methods and techniques that should help to bring the model to life.

## APPLICATION

There are a number of strategies that have evolved from theory, which can be particularly useful when conducting narrative therapy. Within this chapter they are grouped into three processes: getting to know the problem; developing alternative stories; and re-enforcing therapeutic conversations.

### Getting to know the problem (naming/externalising/deconstructing)

From a narrative therapy perspective, problems are constructed by the language available to the person or people experiencing the problem. At times conversations can become so dominated by talk of the problem that there is little room for anything else. This is referred to as a 'thin description' because it lacks the richness of context, complexity and exceptions to the rule that comes with a thickened narrative.

When a person accesses therapy, they often do so with a narrative relating to a problem[1] which encompasses them to the extent that they feel unable to overcome it. The first step for the narrative therapist in beginning to address the power of language in this process is to empower the person to name the problem themselves. For example, one may ask 'What would you call this problem that has led to you being here today?' It can also be helpful to listen out for words that recur; what better way to facilitate a naming of the problem than to ask 'You have used the word X a few times, is that a name you give to the problem?'

This is also where the process of externalising the problem begins. In order to separate the person from the problem, it is referred to as an adjective rather than a noun. For example, one might ask questions such as 'How does the compulsion interfere with your daily life?', 'What effect does the anger have on your relationships?' Notice how the process also involves using 'the' as a prefix to add to the transformation. Adding '-ing' to verbs can also reinforce the externalisation; for example, 'This shouting and hitting' rather than 'When you shout and hit'. Finally, remember to externalise the positive as well as the negative. Not only does this make the whole practice more coherent, also it means that no single account is privileged over another due to social pressures.

Naming the problem, externalising it and generally getting to understand its impact on a person's life can be facilitated by mapping the problem using the 'statement of position' map (White, 2007: 38). White's 'statement of position' map has four components, which may be summarised as follows:

For some great examples of 'maps' and 'charts' to guide narrative therapy conversations, check out White's (2007) *Maps of Narrative Practice*.

1. **Negotiating a particular experience/near definition of the problem:** (Getting to understand how a person makes sense of the problem.) This is the difficult task of finding out what words the person uses in relation to the problem. Mastering this bit will help the rest of the intervention flow quite naturally. Perhaps the most well-known example of this technique is that of 'Sneaky Poo'. This was the name given by a young man to a problem that is commonly referred to by professionals as encopresis (White, 1984).[2]
2. **Mapping the effects of the problem:** Essentially, this is exploring how the problem influences a person's identity. Find out how it affects the person's life in all areas such as at home/work/school, with their family/friends/strangers, and how it makes them think about themselves/their past, present and future.
3. **Evaluating the effects of the problem's activities:** This component is fairly self-explanatory. It is about developing a rich understanding of what techniques the problem uses to assert itself on a person's life, and how that person 'positions' themselves in relation to the effects of the problem. Summarising the conversation presents an opportunity to review the effects of the problem and how they are evaluated. (One word of caution though: avoid 'totalising descriptions'(White, 2007: 34). A totalising

description is one that evaluates the effect of a problem solely in negative terms. Most problems have positive aspects as well.)

4. **Justifying the evaluation:** This is all about the 'Why, of people's evaluations' (White, 2007: 48). The aim of questions in this part of the map is to explore why the person has drawn these specific conclusions about the topic at hand. To some extent, this is the first stage in deconstructing the problem, as we are beginning to explore what has led to its development.

**Example:** An 11-year-old girl was referred to child and adolescent mental health services with 'severe claustrophobia'. This interfered with her family, education and social life. She called the problem the 'What ifs' because she would often state 'What if X happened (e.g. door got stuck, plane crashed, people forgot I was in here)'. As well as causing difficulties, 'What ifs' also helped her avoid some of the many disasters she heard about on the news. Unfortunately it also caused her to be labelled as the 'family worrier'.

Helpful questions in the justifying section included:

'Why do you think the 'What ifs' have come into your life?'
'What has caused you to feel that 'What ifs' can keep you safe?'
'Where do the 'What ifs' fit into what is important to you?'

> If you would like a concrete example of the use of metaphor in narrative therapy, see Carlson's (1998) case example utilising a computer virus metaphor to illustrate how a person reclaimed their life from depression and marijuana.

Hopefully the subtle changes in language utilised in the narrative therapeutic practices outlined above highlight the philosophical link between power and language.

Another technique, which may bolster this understanding further, is the use of metaphor. We frequently use metaphors in our day-to-day conversations, so it is not surprising if they are often brought to the forefront of conversations in narrative therapy.

Metaphors can be drawn from almost any arena, although battle metaphors should generally be avoided where possible. This is because they can increase stress levels, and cause important nuances to be missed (Carey and Russell, 2002). However, whilst battle metaphors should not be introduced by the narrative therapist, if it is the only (or preferred) form of words a person has for referring to the problem, then it would be inattentive to ignore it. After all, the metaphor is:

> only meant to offer a different way to explain how problems work in people's lives and how life stories can be reclaimed.
>
> (Carlson, 1998: 64)

Whilst many of the linguistic/therapeutic tools discussed above are useful in their own right, as a collection they constitute a deconstruction of the problem. Deconstruction involves placing the problem in context; it 'unmasks' oppressive discourses both locally (e.g. within peer and family groups) and more widely (e.g. within the media and in academic texts). All of which helps the person to 'become motivated to deal with problems differently' (Freedman and Coombs, 2005: 68), an outcome that any therapist would value.

## Developing alternative stories (unique outcomes/ thickening the alternative narrative)

Most people access therapy because they want to find a way out of the problem, rather than become more familiar with it. In narrative therapy the two things work in tandem. Becoming more familiar with the problem helps to really understand what has led to it becoming so dominant, what values it is indicative of, and how it is both helpful and a hindrance.

From this platform we can begin to explore how those same values and narratives can be revealing of a life outside of the problem. We delve into (or thicken) times when the problem is less dominant, using similar techniques to those outlined in the previous section. The aim is to create space for alternative stories of the past, present and future to be heard outside of the problem-saturated narrative.

This process begins by looking for exceptions to the rules that govern the problem. These exceptions are often referred to in narrative therapy texts as 'unique outcomes' or 'sparkling moments'. Essentially, they are times when the problem has either not been present or has been less influential over a person's life.

> **Example:** Elijah is a 42-year-old man who has a long-standing diagnosis of depression. In getting to know the problem, Elijah gave it the name 'The Lead Cloud'. At first he felt that 'The Lead Cloud' was always pressing down on him. However, we soon established a sparkling moment that involved an interesting conversation with a librarian. The conversation made Elijah feel valued as a person, and someone with whom others could share an interest with. Elijah could still feel the presence of 'The Lead Cloud', but it was much further away and lighter than he was used to.

Unique outcomes can often be identified without specific forms of questioning. It can be more about the art of listening; trying to hear examples that seem incongruent with the problem narrative. Morgan (2000: 52–3) lists 11 different forms of unique outcomes that include thoughts, plans and beliefs, as well as the more tangible actions and statements. Some examples of questions that can highlight unique outcomes include: 'Are there times when X doesn't seem as prominent?', 'Can you describe a time when you have managed to overcome X even for a short time?' It can also be helpful to frame questions in line with the metaphor; here's a few from conversations with Elijah:

> **Example:** 'Are there times when 'The Lead Cloud' is lighter?'
>
> 'Sometimes I hear on weather forecasts that a strong wind will blow the clouds over quickly, what conditions in your life make 'The Lead Cloud' blow away?'
>
> 'Is there anyone you know who might not notice 'The Lead Cloud' as much as you do?'

Freedman and Combs in particular give plenty of excellent examples, and point out that we should always check that the unique outcomes we are exploring are actually a 'preferred experience' (2005: 92). It is always important in narrative therapy to be aware of our own or societal values.

As therapists we can't help but be curious. It's that curiosity which is the basis of questions that thicken the narrative. There are many narrative therapy texts and maps of narrative practice that will guide you through the process of exploring unique outcomes. However, it is fairly similar to the way you explore the problem. You are looking to bring to life the topic at hand, map its history, influence, helpfulness and hindrances, as well as finding out what it tells us about the values of the person with whom we are conversing. This whole method is referred to as a 're-authoring conversation'.

White (2007) talks about using 'scaffolding questions' as an aid to developing the alternative story. It's not vital to get a grasp on this concept, and it comes with other strange associated terms like 'zones of proximal development'. All it really means is that the questions we use should balance being challenging enough to create space for change, but not so challenging that they alienate the person we are working with. It is the responsibility of the narrative therapist to judge what pace is most useful for the re-authoring conversations. White points out that accepting this responsibility can also help guard against dismissing a person as 'resistant' or 'failing to engage'.

> If you're feeling quite brave by now, have a read of some Vygotsky or Todorov to see where some of this comes from. If you're feeling less brave but want to know a bit more, check out the work of Jerome Bruner (family therapist).

Questions that are paced and framed well can add richness of context to unique outcomes, and give space for a thickening of alternative stories. Some of this can also come from general therapeutic questions that are not model specific. I'm sure we've all said things in therapy along the lines of 'Why is X important to you?', 'I was really struck by you saying …', 'Can you tell me a bit more about …' These are all useful questions to utilise when thickening the alternative story. However, with narrative therapy we are aiming to go a bit deeper and uncover what the person's own interpretation/narrative is. They are, after all, an expert on their own lived stories.

White (2007) refers to the 'landscape of action' and 'landscape of identity (or consciousness)' as helpful concepts for enhancing the alternative story. The landscape of action is what we might refer to as the explicit stuff, for example what happened, where and when, whereas the landscape of identity is more about the implicit, what do we understand about something, what value is it given, and what does it tell us about the internal experience of it. Narrative therapy conversations move freely between these two 'landscapes', with the hope that by exploring a life that is not dominated by the problem, then the problem becomes less dominant.

## Re-enforcing therapeutic conversations (inviting others in/ therapeutic documents)

In most stories there is more than one person involved and a person's narrative is much the same. This section examines some of the practices used in narrative therapy to include others as ways of re-enforcing therapeutic conversations. We also describe methods such as therapeutic documents and definitional ceremonies that can be particularly useful in re-enforcing therapeutic gains. These all serve to increase the impact and sustainability of therapeutic gains.

Remembering conversations are used to give the person we are working with control over who is involved in their newly developed alternative story. The reason being that problem narratives can often lead to 'isolation and disconnection from important relationships' (Morgan, 2000: 77). Therefore, in order to change those patterns, narrative therapy provides an opportunity to invite those important relationships back into a person's life. There are many ways in which to do this, the most obvious of which is to ask the person about the people who are or have been important to them and what they would think of the unique outcomes and alternative story that have been identified.

It is important to note that the figure invited in can be real or imaginary (even pets or toys) and can be from the past, present or future, so they do not have to physically be in the room. Their presence goes some way towards contextualising and emphasising previously subjugated narratives. We can then use scaffolding questions, and maps of narrative practice to thicken the conversations further. Other, perhaps more powerful ways of including those important relationships are to use methods that literally invite them into the room.

> **Example:** Tanya is a 14-year-old girl who experienced 'panic attacks' after being involved in a serious car accident. After developing a sense of strength and control over the attacks and her life she wanted to invite others to witness the impact. So the final therapy session was a party for her friends and family to join her in celebrating her achievements. During the party she gave a speech, in which she told the story of her life and what she valued about their parts in it.

This is an example of what might be termed a 'definitional ceremony', where an audience is invited to hear the story. The audience are referred to as 'outsider witnesses', and their role is to witness and respond with their own acknowledgement. For narrative therapists, it is important that this acknowledgement is not applause in the common sense, as this is loaded with social expectations of what is admirable or otherwise. Instead, we invite them to say what aspects of the story stood out for them and how it relates to their own values.

Another way to enhance the therapeutic process can be to involve 'experience consultants'. These are people who have experienced similar problems to the ones being faced by the person who is currently accessing therapy. It can be incredibly powerful for a person to connect with the words of another person who has shared a similar experience. As you begin using narrative therapy, it is definitely worth asking people if they would be willing to act as experience consultants in the future, and keeping a log of volunteers. However, as always, be ethically and morally sensitive when using this technique.

Most therapy is time-limited, and for the majority of their time a person is not in therapy, therefore we conclude with a tangible way of re-enforcing therapeutic conversations with therapeutic documents. These can take many forms, broadly organised into four groups:

1. **Letters:** These are generally records of the session and may be written at any point, for example after every session, once we have got to know the problem, and then again once the alternative story has been thickened, or as a summary once therapy has come to a close.
2. **Documents of knowledge and affirmation:** These documents focus on the person's preferred identity. They are usually created collaboratively and should be able to be carried around. One form could be a list of the things a person values about themselves and their life. You could even put it on a pocket-sized card and laminate it for extra wear.
3. **News documents:** This is a way of communicating with people who are important to the person (think back to remembering conversations). One example is for the person to write a letter about the alternative story and send it to someone important to them.

4. **Documents to contribute to rites of passage:** These documents are ways of celebrating the gains that have been made during therapy. The most common form is a specially made certificate.

(Adapted from Fox, 2003)

**Example:** For Tanya, who was referred to above, a certificate was presented at the celebration. It was worded in the metaphor she had developed and awarded for 'The Most Valiant Decision to Take Charge of Her Own Life'.

So there we have it, narrative therapy as we have interpreted it. Hopefully it feels accessible and you'll be inspired to incorporate it into your preferred identity. It can be utilised with both children and adults, individuals and groups,[3] and in dealing with any number of problems. We wish you many sparkling moments in its application.

## CASE STUDY

Scott, a 24-year-old male, was referred by his general practitioner for help with managing his anger. This had become particularly intense after he was assaulted on a night out. Scott lived at home with his mother and 19-year-old sister (Amber); he had a long-term girlfriend (Katie), who also spent most nights at Scott's family home.

The initial assessment took place at the family home, with everyone named above in attendance. They presented a consistent story between them, which placed the problem as central to Scott's being, as it defined him in everyone's eyes. Their story briefly summarised was:

Scott's parents had run a pub together until they separated when Scott was approximately 11 years old, after which Scott and Amber moved home with their mother. Things were relatively OK for the next few years, but when Scott was about 15, he started developing 'anger problems'. He would often get into fights, and had a lot of trouble in school. Things calmed down a bit in his late teens, when he met Katie. However, following the assault, he started developing anger problems again. This was mostly in the form of verbal aggression, and mainly towards his mother. There had been a physical element on at least two occasions, one of which resulted in him 'trashing the house' and holding a knife to his mother's throat. All of the family had started to become scared of Scott, and he was becoming more and more withdrawn.

*(Continued)*

*(Continued)*

Scott's relationship with anger actually began when he was living in the pub with his parents. He used to stay up late, and often witnessed incidents of aggression occurring between clientele. Whilst his parents were not violent, they did often have disagreements that led to verbally aggressive arguments. Even when Scott's parents separated, there continued to be arguments between the family, particularly at highly emotional events such as funerals and weddings. Furthermore, there were often fights between his schoolmates as a way of proving their dominance. All in all, Scott said that what he'd learned for sure was that 'The best way to defend is to attack' and that 'You need to be tough to get through life'.

This picture was played out frequently during therapeutic sessions, with regular 'cooling off breaks' required for each of the family members. During an early conversation Scott started to refer to anger as a surge that overcame him, which he had no control over. We started to refer to 'The Surge' in externalising terms. The metaphor seemed to work for Scott, as well as his mother, sister and girlfriend. All of them said that they wished he could take control of 'The Surge' because they found it scary. Scott said that this would be easier if people didn't 'push his buttons' so often. Scott said that his family in particular knew exactly what pushed his buttons.

Button-pushing and surges seemed to present the opportunity of a metaphor relating to electricity. After three sessions the concept was explored via a therapeutic letter to Scott; here's an extract:

> We've discussed the things that have led to 'The Surge' being in your life, and it got me thinking about the challenge being a bit like trying to control electricity, which I guess would make you the electrician. I wonder whether a circuit breaker might be a solution to 'The Surges'? I've enclosed a circuit breaker as a bit of a reminder that there are ways to control 'The Surge'. I was looking for a definition of a circuit breaker and found the following: 'If a power surge occurs in the electrical wiring, the breaker will trip. This means that a breaker which is in the 'on' position will flip to the 'off' position and shut down the electrical power leading from that breaker. Essentially a circuit breaker is a safety device.'

This seemed to be a real turning point for Scott and his family. At the following session, they were all able to give examples from the interim, in which 'The Surge' would have occurred, but didn't.

These examples brought about a discussion where Scott said that the most important thing in his life is his family. He felt that it had been his responsibility to take on the role of 'the man of the house'. Everything he had learned from his experiences taught him that this needed to involve an element of violence. However, this was not Scott's inner belief; he actually felt that if he were to become a father, then he would want his child not to have any violence or aggression in his life. He said that one of the things that had drawn him to Katie was that she 'never went to bed with bad feelings, and never shouted'.

From this Katie told of a time recently when she had been out with Scott, and they had bumped into Amber in the pub. Amber was being 'pestered' by a man she had met. In the past Scott would have 'decked him', but on this occasion he went over to Amber, bought her a drink and invited her to sit with them. By doing so, he created an escape route for Amber that was non-confrontational. Katie said that she was very proud of him for this, and that it was a sign of the kind of man she wanted to marry. This was the first time she had used words such as this and Scott was visibly moved.

Amber said that for her, it was like him 'being a big brother instead of a dad'. There had been many times when she felt he had confused the roles, by 'bossing her around', and that this was what led up to many of their conflicts. Their mother also said that he took on the father role unnecessarily, and conversations about this were often the beginning of arguments between them. In fact, on the occasion when he had held a knife to her throat, the situation had escalated from a discussion about whether or not Amber should be allowed to stay out for the night.

This led to an interesting form of a remembering conversation and a definitional ceremony rolled into one. The family had made the decision not to invite Scott and Amber's father into the sessions, and wanted to maintain that dynamic. However, they were willing to discuss what he would say had he been there, particularly in relation to the situation in the pub with Amber. On from this each person who was present was given a card. Amber's was titled 'What I value about my brother', Katie's 'What I value about my boyfriend', Scott's mother's 'What I value about my son' and Scott's said 'What I value about myself'. These were all completed, and included points such as: he is caring, he understands me, he is honest. The important thing

*(Continued)*

*(Continued)*

was that they valued him as a person, and they were qualities that could reinforce his role as a man, outside of anger, violence and 'The Surge'.

Scott was discharged from the service shortly after this, with a follow-up session six months later. They all attended the follow-up and reported that Scott was 'a changed man'. Whilst 'The Surge' had started on two or three occasions, it had never taken hold. He had been able to flick the switch to 'off'. Scott kept the circuit breaker on his windowsill as a reminder and the cards in his wallet. There had been no further incidents of violence or aggression, despite external incidents that would have instigated it in the past. (See Figure 7.1 for a diagrammatic formulation of scott's case.)

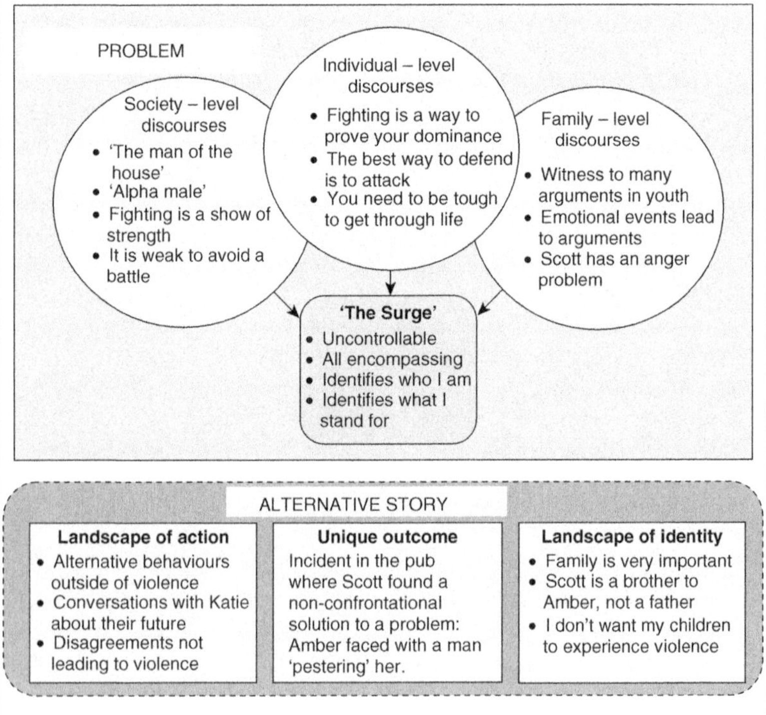


**Figure 7.1** Scott's diagrammatic formulation

## PHILOSOPHY

Hopefully by this point you have gained a reasonable introduction into narrative therapy and ways in which the model can be utilised to help re-shape problematic stories, using techniques such as externalisation, deconstruction and the identification of unique outcomes. However, to fully appreciate the applicability of this model we suggest you take the time to read the following section relating to the philosophical underpinnings of the model. Awareness of this information is important for any therapist wishing to integrate the model into their practice in a well-informed way.

The model is built on poststructuralist philosophy, which grew by way of opposition to the 'structuralist' perspective which developed at the start of the nineteenth century. As the name suggests, structuralism is built on the view that the underlying structures of anything (e.g. language, culture) can be mapped and scientifically investigated. Poststructuralists, on the other hand, argued that the examination of structures is biased and subjective. The 'truth' is not something that can be discovered, instead it is fluid and open to interpretation by individuals and society.

Post-structuralism really came to prominence in the 1960s through leading figures such as Foucault, Derrida, Deleuze and Lyotard. They analysed their own and others' texts on subjects including philosophy, psychology and anthropology, written by people such as Kant, Neitzche and Freud. Poststructuralist philosophy has had such a big (and controversial) impact that it is often discussed in relation to a much earlier period of philosophical riches: The Enlightenment.[4] During the enlightenment era, a number of now familiar concepts were developed, such as rationality, free will and modernity.

These concepts do not sit comfortably with poststructuralism, which argues that societal discourses hold the power to shape and boundary us all in actions and interactions. Poststructuralists see the age of enlightenment as an 'unfinished heritage' (Davies, 2003: 34). They believe that by thoroughly evaluating any assumption, that assumption can be challenged and potentially changed. Reflections on knowledge, language and power are woven into their primary works, with the premise that all forms of knowledge are both limited and limiting. This is particularly noticeable in the works of the two French poststructuralist philosophers, Michel Foucault and Jacques Derrida, who are the focus of our brief foray into philosophy.

### Foucault

Of the poststructuralist philosophers, Michel Foucault is the one most frequently referred to within narrative therapy. Michael White, the person who has had the biggest impact in narrative therapy, specifically highlights the writings of Foucault (White and Epston, 1990; White, 2007), as a major influence on his own practice. Indeed, the opening chapter of *Narrative Means to Therapeutic Ends* is given over to the role of Foucault's work in overcoming what he sees as the 'impasse' between perceptions of power either as an entity in its own right, or as a construction of language (White and Epston, 1990: 1).

Foucault's perspective on the interaction between knowledge and power is an intrinsic part of narrative therapy. In Besley's (2001) reflections on the work of Michael White and David Epston, she highlights four main aspects of how Foucauldian thinking on this subject has directly influenced the practice of narrative therapy:

1. **Orientation in therapy:** This means acknowledging that therapy is not apolitical. To do so, therapists must 'demystify' their practices and be aware of their role in knowledge–power dynamics. For narrative therapists, it also means being explicit with the poststructuralist stance on which the approach is built.
2. **Separating from the unitary knowledges:** Poststructuralism argues that there is no truth, no statement, no perspective that is stable, permanent and objective. Everything relies on language and beliefs to hold it in place, all of which are open to challenge.
3. **Challenging the techniques of power:** This is to identify who or what is exercising power in relation to the issue at hand and how that position is maintained. By observing and analysing the processes at play, one can also identify ways to oppose it.
4. **Resurrecting the subjugated knowledges:** Poststructuralists would argue that the positivist view of stable, true knowledge serves to subjugate (marginalise) alternative knowledges. These alternative knowledges can be categorised into those that have been previously known but suppressed, and those that are culturally specific, but are repressed because they do not conform to the dominant discourse.

(Adapted from Besley, 2001)

The work of Foucault is inherent to, but perhaps slightly implicit within, the narrative therapy approach. As one grows more familiar with the language and practice of the model, the previously esoteric nature of Foucault's work also becomes more familiar. It is interesting that this familiarity grows through a grasp of the language, given the emphasis poststructuralists place on language (particularly in relation to knowledge and power). Interestingly, whilst Foucault is mentioned more but his language used less in narrative therapy, our next philosopher, Derrida, is referred to less but his language is used more, particularly with reference to metaphors and 'deconstruction'.

## Derrida

Derrida's thinking and subsequent work was primarily built on his textual analysis, which crossed the borders of subject and included, amongst others, the works of Levi-Strauss, Freud, Rousseau and indeed his friend Foucault. In his deconstruction of both factual and fictional texts, Derrida also drew heavily on the use of metaphors by many of the leading historical and contemporary figures. He argues that the use of metaphors has been central to discourse, and that this is not merely a device to dress-up texts but is central to them (Hepburn, 2000).

Michael White states that metaphors are an important part of narrative therapy conversations because:

> [metaphors] are borrowed from particular discourses that evoke/invoke specific understandings of life and identity.
>
> (2007: 31)

He presents a variety of examples of their usage during externalising conversations, which include ones drawn from diverse sources such as the maritime world, civil action and puppetry (2007: 32–33).

Similarly, examples of another direct impact of Derrida's work, deconstruction, can also be found in core narrative therapy texts. For example, Alice Morgan's 'easy-to-read introduction' to narrative therapy offers six pages to its discussion. She refers to it as 'situating the problem in context', a practice that is hopefully familiar to all therapists.

Derrida coined the term 'deconstruction' (1982), and for him it could be applied to any subject in any format, although he was primarily concerned with text. His view being that no text, no premise, no belief, is true and stable. If you deconstruct anything with enough analytical vigour, then you inevitably undermine its position as an unshakeable entity and replace it with an endless number of alternative possibilities. Within narrative therapy specifically, deconstruction is an overt technique and refers to the process of unpicking the politics of any given problem. The theory, as drawn from Derrida's concept of deconstruction, is that problematic stories can be 'taken apart', or deconstructed. As a consequence, the foundations on which those problems are built can be analysed, evaluated and adapted.

Finally, a quote from *The Oxford Handbook of Political Theory* provides a great example of how the philosophy relates to practice: 'Derrida insists that deconstruction seeks to intervene in order to change things' (Patton, 2006: 126). After all, isn't intervening in order to change things (hopefully for the better) the lifeblood of therapy?

## GLOSSARY

| | |
|---|---|
| Alternative story | Bringing together unique outcomes and thickened descriptions to form a new narrative. |
| Deconstruction | Unpicking the conditions that cause the problem to be overwhelming. |
| Discourse | Conversation(s) laden with both explicit and implicit values. |
| Experience consultants | People who have faced a similar problem in the past and can talk to others who face that problem now. |
| Exploring problem effects | Talking about how the problem has influenced a person's sense of self, thoughts, feelings, relationships, social situation and other aspects of their life. |
| Externalising conversations | Ways of speaking that separate the person's identity from the problem. |
| Landscape of action | Descriptions of the visible, explicit aspects of a story. The what, where and when. |
| Landscape of identity | Descriptions of the internal, implicit aspects of a story. The values, understanding and experience of it. |
| Maps of narrative practice | Guides developed by narrative therapists, predominantly Michael White, to describe the processes and types of questions used in narrative therapy. |
| Outsider witnesses | People who are invited by the person who has accessed therapy to listen to their story. |
| Positivism | The pure scientific stance that exists in pursuit of truths, hypothesis testing and quantitative data production. |
| Poststructuralism | A philosophical perspective that views knowledge, language and power as inextricably linked. |
| Remembering conversations | Using significant relationships as a recruited audience to reinforce new narrative. |
| Scaffolding | Using questions to help a person move from a problem narrative to an alternative story. |
| Sparkling moments | See Unique outcomes |
| Subjugated knowledge | Ideas, beliefs, values or experiences that have been marginalised by discussions overly focused on the problem. |
| Therapeutic documents | Anything tangible outside the therapeutic conversation that is part of the therapeutic process. Examples may include letters, certificates, cards of acknowledgment. |
| Thickening the plot | Enriching the new story and making it feel significant by adding context, meaning and detail. |
| Thin descriptions | Meanings reached in the face of adversity that allow little space for the contradictions of life. Thin descriptions lead to thin conclusions about a person's identity. |
| Totalising descriptions | Descriptions that view any issue in a wholly positive or wholly negative frame. |

| | |
|---|---|
| Tracing the problem's history | Assessing the influence the problem has had in a person's life over time. |
| Unique outcomes | Times when the problem has had little or no influence over an individual. It can be anything that does not fit with the dominant story. |
| Zones of proximal development | The area between what we know now and what we are about to learn. |

## REFERENCES


Besley, T. (2001) 'Foucauldian influences on narrative therapy: An approach for schools', *Journal of Educational Enquiry, 2*, 72–93.

Carey, M. and Russell, S. (2002) 'Externalising: Commonly asked questions', *International Journal of Narrative Therapy and Community Work, 2*, 76–84.

Carlson, T. (1998) 'The virus metaphor and narrative therapy' *The Journal of Family Psychotherapy, 9*, 63–8.

Davies C. (2003) *After Poststructuralism: Reading, Stories and Theory*. London: Routledge.

Derrida, J. (1982) *Margins of Philosophy*. Chicago, IL: University of Chicago Press.

Fox, H. (2003) 'Using therapeutic documents: A review', *International Journal of Narrative Therapy and Community Work, 4*, 26–36.

Freedman, J. and Coombs, G. (2005) *Narrative Therapy: The Social Construction of Preferred Realities*. London: Norton.

Hepburn, A. (2000) 'Power lines: Derrida, discursive psychology and the management of accusations of teacher bullying', *British Journal of Social Psychology, 39*, 605–628.

Morgan, A. (2000) *What is Narrative Therapy?: An Easy to Read Introduction*. Adelaide: Dulwich Centre Publications.

Patton, P. (2006) *The Oxford Handbook of Political Theory* (pp. 125–142). Oxford: Oxford University Press.

Tomm, K. (1989) 'Externalizing the problem and internalizing personal agency', *Journal of Strategic and Systemic Therapies, 8*, 54–59.

Vassallo, T. (2002) 'Narrative therapy with the seriously mentally ill: A case study'. Available at: www.narrativeapproaches.com/narrative%20papers%20folder/mentalill.htm. Originally published in *The Australian and New Zealand Journal of Family Therapy, 19*. (Last accessed 27 August 2011)

White, M. (1984) 'Pseudoencopresis: From avalanche to victory, from vicious to virtuous cycles', *Journal of Family Systems Medicine, 2*, 2150–2160.

White, M. (2007) *Maps of Narrative Practice*. Lodon: Norton.

White, M. and Epston, D. (1990) *Narrative Means to Therapeutic Ends*. London: Norton.


## NOTES

1. This is, of course, assuming that they have been autonomous, or at least in agreement with the process.
2. For a good description of the Sneaky Poo example see the original article, and to see how this relates to wider theory, see Tomm (1989).
3. We haven't given specific examples of using narrative therapy with groups, but there are some good ones out there (e.g. Vassallo, 2002).
4. The Enlightenment period spans the late-seventeenth and eighteenth centuries. Major figures related to the period include Denis Diderot, Immanuel Kant and Rene Descartes.

## Worksheet 7.1

## Getting to know the problem

### The Person is not the Problem, the Problem is the Problem

The first stage in narrative therapy is to get to know the problem and how it has affected a person's life. Remember to frame questions in a manner that externalises the problem and use the language of the person who is accessing therapy. Here are some questions that might be helpful.

- What do you call the problem (X) that led to you being here today?
- How long has X been present in your life?
- What strategies does X use to influence your life?
- Are there times when X can be useful?
- What goals do you think X has?
- Who or what helps X in its mission to achieve those goals?
- What effect has X had on your view of yourself?
- What is the best thing about X?
- What is the worst thing about X?
- Why is it important to you to speak with me about X?
- What are your views on your relationship with X?
- If you were to draw X, what would it look like?
- If you could interview X, what questions would you ask?
- What influence has X had on your life?
- Who else is aware of X?
- What would you imagine to be X's likes and dislikes?
- What have you learned about X in the time X has been in your life?

## Worksheet 7.2

## Developing alternative stories

The trick to developing an alternative story/narrative is to find an example of a time when the problem is not as influential on a person's life. Explore this example in great detail and thicken the narrative around it. Make certain this unique outcome is one that the person values and then facilitate the development of a narrative that is not wholly consumed by the problem. Try using the following guide during a therapy session.

1. Identify a unique outcome
   - Highlight an example of the person's behaviour/values/beliefs/intentions that does not fit with the problem narrative. This may even be a situation where the problem is less dominant.
   - Check that this is a preferred way of being for the person.
2. Thicken this narrative and ascribe meaning to it
   - Consider the landscape of action. Find out about the tangible aspects of the story. What exactly happened? What preparation took place? Who else was involved? When and where did this all occur?
   - Consider the landscape of identity. Find out about the implicit aspects of the story. What is important to the person to allow this to occur? What does it say about their beliefs and values? What does it show about their hopes for the future? What was their personal experience of it?
3. Infuse this into the person's wider narrative
   - Find out about other examples from the past, present and future intentions that are akin to what has been discussed in 1 and 2 above. Explore the landscapes of action and identity in relation to these other examples.

# Worksheet 7.3

## Re-enforcing therapeutic conversations

This next set of questions is commonly used in outsider witness practices in narrative therapy; however, they have much wider applicability. For example, if you are providing a consultation to another professional, you could use the questions to uncover what is important to them about the issue at hand. Another example could be when providing supervision, where they could be used to explore the supervisee's experience of a therapeutic session or service issue. The possibilities are endless, but here's the very simple four-point exploration:

1. **What stood out for you?** Find out what sticks out in the other person's mind/memory when they think back on the issue being discussed.
2. **What image does this invoke?** Encourage the person to develop an image/metaphor that represents what stood out for them in 1 above.
3. **What value does this hook into?** The thing that stood out in 1 above is likely to have done so because it relates to a particular value of theirs: Find out what it is.
4. **Where has this taken you?** Facilitate a discussion about what has changed as a result of the issue at hand. This may be related specifically to the value identified in 3 above, or a more general change. The change may be further embedded by continuing its discussion using the imagery brought out in 2 above.

**Worksheet 7.4**

# *Certificate of Recognition*

*This is to certify that*

____________________

*Has been presented withthe award for*

______________________________

______________________________

*Date* *Presented by*

__________

# 8 PERSON-CENTRED THERAPY

Sharon Twigg

Person-centred therapy (PCT) was developed by Carl Rogers in the early 1940s. The theory was distinguished from other approaches of the time by its non-directive method. The approach trusts that the person accessing therapy will find their own solutions and understandings of their difficulties. Despite a number of changes to the model through the years, the central aim remains: to increase each person's awareness of their deeper feelings, true thoughts and inner resources. This leads to trust in a person's decision making and enables independent problem-solving. The therapist is a 'facilitator' of the process and the individual is central to their own therapy, hence 'person-centred therapy.'

## THE MODEL

### The main principle

In order to understand the complexities of person-centred therapy (PCT), we must first understand the main principle behind the approach as defined by Carl Rogers. He believed that humans are inherently 'good'. By this Rogers meant that each individual will automatically do the best they can with the knowledge or resources they have.

Despite the wonderfully straightforward beliefs on which PCT is built, the approach does contain some confusing terms (e.g. referring to a person as an organism). Most of the terms are defined in the glossary at the end of the chapter; however, 'self-actualising tendency' and 'organismic valuing processes' are particularly unusual but central to the approach (see Table 8.1).

PCT's core principle is that with the right social and psychological environment, a person will blossom. The drive towards becoming the best person we can is known as the 'self-actualising tendency'. Rogers described it as:

| Term | Description | Examples |
|---|---|---|
| Self-actualising tendency | The drive to become the best person we can, in all ways. | Depending on how we are nurtured, we may grow to feel that we can be successful, happy or satisfied. Alternatively, we may believe we are destined for sadness and pain. |
| Organismic valuing processes | Something inside us that gives value ratings to the experiences we have. | Each individual finds that they enjoy or feel comfortable in certain settings, whilst disliking or feeling sad in others. |

**Table 8.1** The two terms central to PCT

> The tendency of the organism [the person] to maintain itself, to assimilate food, to behave defensively in the face of threat, to achieve the goal of self-maintenance even when the usual pathway to that goal is blocked … The tendency of the organism to move in the direction of maturation, as maturation is defined for each species.
>
> (Rogers, 1951: 488)

Rogers believed that this tendency was so strong that only death can stop it. However, it can be stunted by negative influences or limited resources. This is why children who suffered negative experiences such as neglect or abuse may be developmentally inhibited, but once given the right support can still blossom.

## Internal valuing system – the needs of the individual

As well as a person's self-actualising tendency, Rogers believed that every individual has an internal valuing system that helps to place a value rating on everyday things. For example, we may think of them as likeable, safe, threatening or comfortable. These ratings are unique to each individual and known in PCT as the 'organismic valuing processes'.

From birth, a person's organismic valuing processes are directly linked to their newly developing self-actualising tendency. For an example, see Figure 8.1.

## The effects of others, external stimuli and the environment

An infant's development relies heavily on its parent's response. A lack of resources, such as a shortage of food or a parent's lack of nurturing, will have a significant impact on a young child. Therefore, the surrounding conditions and actions of a child are highly important in shaping a child's self-actualising tendency. For example, a parent who ignores their child's cries for hunger will influence their child's behaviour. Either the child will stop its efforts or it will cry louder in an attempt to get its needs met by the parent.

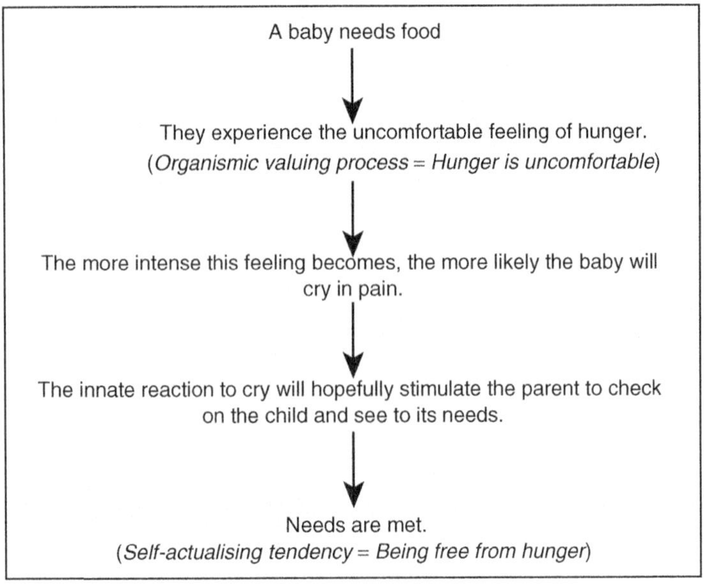


**Figure 8.1** The developing process from birth

Rogers believed that with the right parental support a child could adjust to the competing demands of their environment without inhibiting their self-actualising tendency or dismissing their organismic valuing processes. This is thought to be most evident when a parent's response of displeasure towards a child's behaviour (e.g. throwing food) also manages to acknowledge the child's internal experience (e.g. 'I'm happy, throwing food is fun!') and developmental stage (e.g. 'Hey, I can throw pretty well!'). Therefore, a child is always positively and unconditionally loved as well as encouraged to develop the best they can.

Over time, the infant begins to understand itself through other's responses, and eventually develops a perception of themselves (their *self-concept*). This self-concept may be negative or positive, depending on how others have regarded the child. Therefore, how a child is treated will affect how they see themselves, and how well they function as a person.

> According to Rogers, during infancy the child learns to adjust their behaviour to fit with their environment. This inevitably impacts on their self-actualising tendency (Saunders, 2006).

Furthermore, Rogers (1961) suggests that a 'fully functioning' person must have experienced three nurturing key factors from their parents:

- Unconditional acceptance (you are accepted for all that you are).
- Unconditional regard (you are loved whatever you do).
- Unconditional approval (you will always be supported).

In such a supportive environment, a child will continue to connect with their organismic valuing processes, whilst adapting to their social environment and developing towards their self-actualising tendency.

Moreover, the early messages received from their parents (e.g. 'I am loved' or 'I am unwanted') becomes part of the child's understanding of how they are 'valued'. This concept will in turn shape how they value themselves. For example, does the child come to understand they are 'mummy's little treasure', or second to the family cat? Eventually, this value will become part of our self-concept, known as our *self-worth*.

Depending on the earlier life experiences, a person's perception and value of themselves may be healthy, damaged or inaccurate. Furthermore, these perceptions will influence what a person considers their self-actualising tendency to be. A positive concept may promote the perception that 'the world is my oyster', while a negative concept may inhibit them to believe something along the lines of 'I will always be second best so why bother?'.

The key thing to remember in PCT is that a good balance of the components of 'the selves' is important to maintain and promote a healthy individual. Figure 8.2 illustrates the linking of all the parts of the selves.

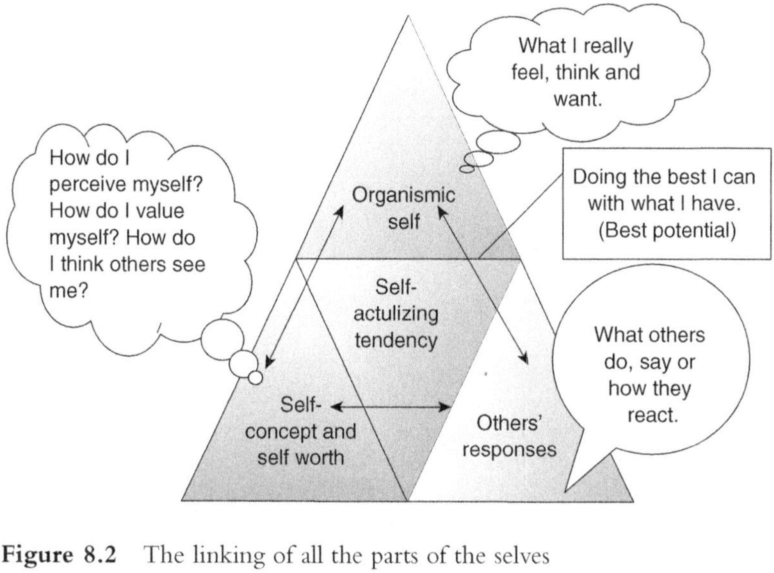


**Figure 8.2** The linking of all the parts of the selves

The role of therapy and the therapist according to PCT is to support a person in becoming a 'fully functioning adult' (i.e. one who has a good perception and value of themselves). This is done by helping them to bring together the component parts of their selves. Rogers (1961) believed that a fully functioning adult would:

- Be open to experiences.
- Embrace each experience and accept change.
- Have trust in their inner thoughts, feeling and reactions.
- Understand that they determine and control their behaviour rather than believing that others have this power.

If a person manages to achieve this, then they should be true to their feelings, thoughts and reactions. They should also have a realistic take on who they are as a person (a real self). It is important to also say that they can still hold an idea of who they would like to become (an ideal self), whilst they acknowledge and accept themselves as they are. The greater the overlap between the two states of self, the greater the 'congruence' (see Figure 8.3).

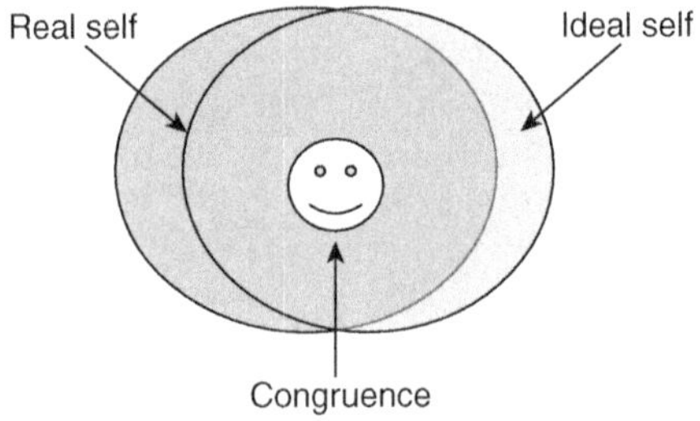


**Figure 8.3** Achieving congruence

In essence, a positive self-concept and self-worth allows a person to trust in their inner thoughts and feelings. This promotes development towards our old friend: self-actualising tendency. The individual will then be more likely to understand themselves and their world through their own experiences, rather than through others' expectations or demands.

## Incongruence (the not so fully functioning person)

In contrast with congruence, Rogers (1961) referred to an imbalanced state of wellbeing as 'incongruence'. This occurs when a person's self-concept and self-worth are heavily based on how others see them. This inevitably results in their own organismic valuing processes being played down. It typically occurs when an individual has had conditions placed on the love or feeling of worth they receive. For example, a parent may give the conditional message that 'daddy only loves you when you are good'. This shapes the belief that love is conditional and can be withdrawn. The child may then put effort into meeting the demands of the parent to receive consistent love, while ignoring their inner feelings (which may be frustration or sadness).

Furthermore, such conditions may lead an individual to developing a self-concept that is selective. For example, they may only acknowledge the certain organismic valuing processes that are considered acceptable, while rejecting others that are not. Trust in the person's own real thoughts and feelings can become weakened by the drive to become the ideal self. The result is a relatively small overlap between the real self and the ideal self (see Figure 8.4).

> Issues of incongruence experienced by the therapist should be discussed in supervision, and if appropriate reflected with the person (Tolan, 2003).

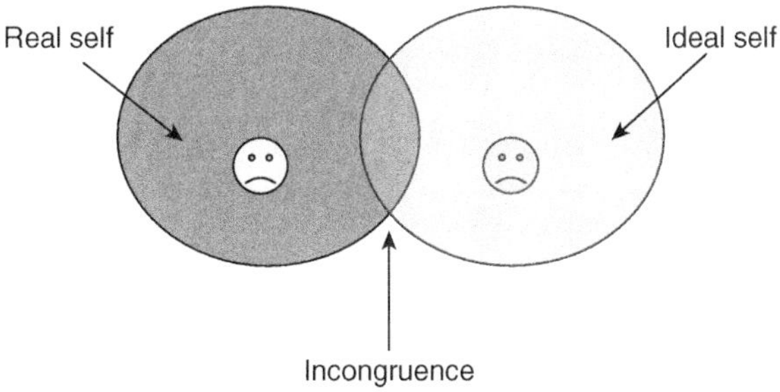


**Figure 8.4** Selective self-concept leads to incongruence

## The person in therapy

Individuals who experience an incongruent state of self are seen as being torn between their 'real' and 'ideal' selves. In order to meet the concept of the ideal self, the person may put a lot of effort into hiding the true thoughts or feelings of the real self. They become focused on what they think they should be, rather than simply being who they are. This can often be observed in a person's language, for example they may frequently use phrases such as 'I ought to ...', 'I should ...', and 'I can't ...'.

However, given the nature of society, we are all subject to conditions being placed on our experiences. These may make us often feel as though our needs are not being met, and may also slightly restrict our self-actualising tendency. We may find ourselves in certain situations where we feel obliged to meet external conditions to get what we need. For example, we may wear our hair differently speak, differently and hide our fear during a job interview.

We are all likely to have developed an ideal self at some point in our lives. What really matters is the size of overlap between the real and ideal self. In therapy we aim to promote a good deal of overlap. Indeed, Rogers believed that the greater the distance between the real and ideal self, the more the self will be fractured. Thus, the more likely a person will suffer emotional distress. Many people who seek therapeutic support are often at this state of being.

At the heart of the therapeutic process lies the goal of helping a person acknowledge the fracture between the real and ideal self. From there we can help a person discover 'who' they are in the absence of unhelpful demands from others. Roger's (1959) strongly believed that only then can a person begin to fully recognise themselves and their inner resources. Acknowledging these resources would then help them to heal the fractured parts, and form a healthy perception of their self.

## APPLICATION

Unlike in many other models, PCT therapists do not tend to start with a series of questions about the person, such as those regarding their childhood, problems, status and history. Instead, it is trusted that what is important to the person will be brought by them naturally. The therapist simply facilitates the process using the six core conditions (see below). Relevant experiences will always be raised by the person if they are important enough.

Furthermore, while the person accessing therapy may make significant efforts to remain distant from their real self, the PCT approach holds faith that a person will always reveal their organismic valuing processes. For example in the dialogue below, despite Mary's best efforts to ignore her 'silly' teary outburst, the real feelings of sadness cannot be pushed aside forever.

**Example:**

*Mary*: I don't know what's wrong with me. I keep bursting into tears at the slightest silly thing. [*Mary cries but quickly dabs her tears away*]

*Therapist*: You sound frightened, like this is something you've never experienced before.

*Mary*: I am! I mean I haven't cried since I was 5. Crying doesn't solve anything!

*Therapist*: But now it seems like you don't have a choice.

*Mary*: Yes, like all those tears have been stored up over the years and now they are flooding out.

*Therapist*: Hmmm, that's a lot of stored up tears.

*Mary*: [*Mary goes quiet in thought*] Maybe they aren't so silly; I mean 40 years without crying can't be that good for you, but we weren't encouraged to cry.

## Main aim (facilitating therapy)

Instead of directing therapy, the PCT therapist aims to provide a climate that facilitates therapeutic change. This climate is similar to a nurturing parent (remember those three needs from before?):

For a personal account regarding therapeutic facilitation and the fundamental principles of PCT, read Chapter 2 in Rogers (1961).

- Unconditional acceptance.
- Unconditional regard.
- Unconditional approval.

In addition, facilitation may be reflected within the set-up of the therapy room. Typically, PCT is conducted with little more than two chairs spaced equally apart and at a slight angle (often 45 degrees), so that each does not face each other directly. This is important for engagement and to avoid each feeling their personal space is being invaded. It also gives the person accessing therapy, the 'visual space' to look away from the therapist while remaining engaged. This may be helpful during uncomfortable feelings, such as embarrassment, or reflective periods of thought.

Furthermore, no desk, coffee table or giant-sized plant should obstruct the space between the two persons, as these are potential barriers between each person. Instead, the open setting aims to facilitate 'openness to the experience' by the two individuals involved.

Often the therapist will wait for the client to get themselves comfortable before starting the session. They may reflect on their own feelings as well as what the person might be feeling, for example 'I find it a bit tense at first meeting new people and you may be feeling the same'. The therapist may then go on to begin the session, such as 'Have you had PCT counselling before' or 'Would it help to explain a little of what we will be doing?', or:

> This is a space for you to talk about what you feel is important to you. I am no expert and I do not have the answers to your difficulties, but together we can explore the experiences you bring each session. Maybe together we can find the answers you are looking for which I believe lie within you. While I will be accepting of what you tell me I will also reflect on my experience of you and what I might be thinking, observing or feeling. Do you have any questions or do you feel ready to talk about what has brought you here today?

However, facilitation of therapy can only work if the person is in a position of incongruence (Mearns and Thorne, 2007; Saunders, 2006). Rogers (1959) suggested therefore that six core conditions are necessary for therapy to work.

### The six core conditions

1. **Psychological contact**: The therapist and the person are in psychological contact (Rogers, 1959). In other words, the person and the therapist are aware that their feelings, presence or beliefs will have an impact on each other and the relationship.
2. **Person's incongruence**: The person is in an incongruent position (as explained previously).
3. **Therapist's congruence**: The therapist is in a congruent position. Therefore, the therapist is honest and genuine with the person and takes on the role of a facilitator to the therapy rather than an 'expert', 'teacher' or 'leader'.
4. **Unconditional positive regard**: The therapist experiences unconditional positive regard for the person and communicates this to the person. For this to happen, the therapist must encourage a person to explore their thoughts and feelings without the threat of rejection, criticism or judgement.
5. **Empathic understanding**: The therapist experiences empathic understanding and focuses on understanding the person's experience, feelings or thoughts. The therapist reflects this understanding back to the person while communicating the value of the person's view and experience.
6. **Clear communication**: The therapist maintains clear communication, unconditional positive regard and empathic understanding to facilitate change.

Although this may seem like a tall order for therapists to achieve in every session, Rogers (1961) points out that therapists are only human, therefore they are likely to experience incongruence from time to time. They may also struggle to like every person they work with because, as Mearns (1994) points out, liking and unconditional positive regard do not go hand in hand.

## Therapist's personal style and reflections

True to the nature of PCT, the personal style of each therapist will influence the therapy they deliver. The style will influence their reflections, which communicate their congruence towards the person. Over time, the therapist's reflections will become more natural and observant. For example, in Joe's therapy below, the therapist facilitated Joe's connection to his feelings. By reflecting upon Joe's body language, facial expression and using word-for-word reflection, Joe begins to 'hear' himself.

**Example:**

*Joe*: I am so confused right now I feel like I could scream!

*Therapist*: I really hear how distressing this confusion is for you. You're holding your hands by your mouth and look like you could just 'scream' it right out.

*Joe*: I get so … so … I don't know [*clenches fist and grits teeth*].

*Therapist*: [*Pause*] You look like you might be also feeling … angry? You're all balled up, fists clenched and teeth gritted.

*Joe*: Not angry. I'm furious!

In the above example, the therapist communicates what they have heard the person say, as well as what they have seen in the person's behaviour or actions. This is reflected carefully, and without judgement or expert opinions. It should then help the person connect to their real self.

## The process of therapy

Rogers (1951) believed in the natural process of PCT where therapeutic change would always happen at some level for the person. The existence of all six core conditions was essential to set a process of therapy in motion. This process was thought to have 12 characteristic directions as in Table 8.2.

If a therapist does not engage fully (i.e. put effort into developing a genuine therapeutic relationship) or provide the core conditions, change is expected to be minimal (Rogers, 1959). Therefore, the therapist's skill of facilitation is imperative for the process to work.

Although much of the therapy process involves the skills of the therapist, it should be noted that the stage at which a person enters into therapy is equally important. Rogers (1961) believed that there may be times when a person is at a stage in their lives where they are not ready to engage in therapy, despite a therapist's best efforts to support them with the process

> For an interesting account of the person's stages of process, have a read of Chapter 7 in Rogers (1961), or a 'nutshell' version in Casemore, Chapter 5 (2006).

## Therapy, timing and reviews

It is not typical to time constrain the number of sessions offered to a person due to the 'person-led' approach. However, in reality a therapist may be bound by logistical constraints. Brief PCT is achievable, and details of this can be seen in Mearns (1994) and Mearns and Thorne (1988).

If brief counselling is offered, the therapist must assess beforehand if this is appropriate for the person. For example, vulnerable people may struggle to end

| | |
|---|---|
| 1. | The person is free to express their feelings verbally or behaviourally. |
| 2. | These feelings give reference to the person's real self as they become more in touch with their inner feelings, thoughts and reactions. |
| 3. | The person increasingly differentiates and discriminates between their feelings and imposed perceptions from others, the environment and experiences. The person becomes aware of the links between these areas of the self and begins to experience things more accurately. |
| 4. | Expressed feelings increase the incongruence between what they feel and their current self-concept. |
| 5. | The person fully experiences the threat of such incongruence. This is supported by the therapist's unconditional positive regard. |
| 6. | The person fully experiences feelings from the past that may have been denied, distorted or out of awareness. |
| 7. | The person's self-concept begins to include these felt experiences which were previously denied. |
| 8. | Reorganisation of the self-structure continues and the self-concept becomes increasingly congruent through this experience. The person will now recognise experiences that were once too threatening to acknowledge. The person's defensiveness decreases as they become more open to experience. |
| 9. | The person is increasingly able to experience, without a felt threat, the therapist's unconditional positive regard. |
| 10. | The person continually feels an unconditional regard for themselves. |
| 11. | The person increasingly puts trust in their inner resources to evaluate their experiences. |
| 12. | The person reacts to experiences in terms of their true self rather than the conditions of worth. |

**Table 8.2** The 12 characteristic directions of PCT (adapted from Rogers, 1959)

an in-depth therapeutic relationship, and may well feel abandoned at discharge (Saunders, 2006). To avoid this, a therapist may help a person prepare for the ending of therapy by raising it early on in their work together, for example 'Do you have any ideas when it might be an appropriate time to stop therapy?'

Mearns and Thorne (1988, 2007) suggest that a review of the therapeutic process may help a person to understand their progress within the process of therapy. For example, Stacey accessed PCT and when reflecting on her experience said: 'We just seemed to talk a lot and then like a jigsaw puzzle the pieces of me fell into place. I don't know when it happened, but I can see how far I have come.'

In addition, a therapist may be advised to discuss reviews or restarts of therapy, so that a person is not misguided into thinking that PCT therapy is a one-off engagement. However, follow-up sessions are not compulsory to the approach, as each therapist holds faith in the person's best potential. They hold faith that a person will continue to do the best for themselves and become the person they truly want to be. For example, Mike struggled to accept that he had assets that made him a good friend. However, with therapy he had learned to accept some of the real feelings and thoughts he held:

**Example:** *Mike*: I guess one big change is that I can now accept friend's compliments. Before, I would throw them back or question them. It's almost nice to hear them actually.

*Therapist*: I'm hearing a big change for you is accepting compliments from friends and that this is almost nice. You know you smile when you say that.

*Mike*: I do, don't I? I guess I'm more OK with me than I give myself credit for.

By this acknowledgment, Mike is likely to remain in touch with his experiences and would continue to grow following therapeutic closure.

So, there you have PCT from a start point of understanding some of the challenging terminology used, through to an end point of dealing with therapeutic closure. PCT can be quite difficult to get used to as a model of therapy. However, if we keep its aims and the process central, and acknowledge our own individual take on life and therapy, it can be a very acknowledging way of working.

## CASE STUDY

### Background

Tess was a 25-year-old professional sales person. She was successful in her job and happily married until three years ago when she became 'stressed' and reported feeling unhappy most of the time, which brought her to therapy looking for answers.

### The beginning of the therapeutic process

During the first session, Tess seemed overly 'professional' (a dominant part of her ideal self) and made very clear demands on the therapist. At the same time the therapist noted how inhibited and dislocated Tess was from her inner feelings. The tricky task for the

*(Continued)*

*(Continued)*

therapist was to provide a congruent beginning, whilst trying to address Tess's demands without threat.

*Tess:* [*After hearing the therapist's introduction to PCT*] I thought I could come here today, see an expert and get some guidance on why I'm unhappy! *[Tess shouts].* What's the point of seeing an expert if you're not going to provide me with answers?

*Therapist:* [*Therapist remains calm*]. You came, hoping for answers or guidance and now your visit feels pointless and I can see you're angry about it. [*Pause*] But maybe together we can try to find a way forward or get some clarity of the problem.

As can be seen above, the therapist did not get drawn into a power struggle and remained confident in the process. For Tess, this experience challenged her state of being as she was neither having her demands met nor did she have the answers at hand. After much discussion, Tess decided to continue therapy 'as a trial'.

Following this initial session, the therapist sought supervision to discuss the pressure felt upon them to 'perform' and 'provide answers'. This was kept in mind for the following sessions as the therapist wondered if this was transference of Tess's experience and whether Tess also felt external pressures/conditions to 'perform'.

Further sessions revealed conditions of worth which Tess had grown up with. Many of these conditions stemmed from her parents and seemed related to the pressure 'to perform' (like that felt by the therapist). These conditions included:

- You are good if you are successful (i.e. married, children, nice car, good job).
- You are unlovable if you are a loser.
- You are good if you do what mummy and daddy tell you to.
- You are unforgivable if you hurt mummy or daddy's feelings.
- You are good if you are loving and caring.

Several of these conditions had become so consuming for Tess that an ideal self had become much of her focus in life. For example, Tess believed that to be a successful wife she ought to have had children. This would no doubt please her parents and envy her peers, but was this something Tess wanted?

Furthermore, Tess believed that she needed promotion to show she was 'winning' at work in the face of colleague competition.

Even her 'loving and caring' abilities relied on the success of running charity events or how much money she raised. All this focus lessened the connection to her real feelings, deeper thoughts and inhibited her experiences. For Tess, her real feelings were repressed because this revealed a 'weak, vulnerable and softer' part of herself.

Trusting in the process of therapy, the therapist encouraged Tess to talk. This was done by using reflection, gentle prompts and avoiding putting pressure on Tess which she may experience as pressure to perform.

After a couple of sessions, Tess let down the mask of the 'professional'. She began to talk and cry about the difficulties she was experiencing at work. In the absence of external conditions of worth and being judged as unsuccessful, unlovable or a loser, Tess began to express her true feelings. Tess was experiencing a safe place to let down her guard and connect to her real self.

As a woman in the working world, Tess described the discrepancies she felt between trying to be a successful business person and a wife. This was often experienced in contrast to being a shrewd business woman. She became aware of how unhappy she felt in her job and how frustrated she felt with the external pressure from her loved ones.

Tess also came to realise that much of her unhappiness was caused by her need for perfection. Tess's drive towards becoming her ideal self was unrealistic. The pressure had become too much when she started a new job in a well-known company following her marriage. On top of this, her family's expectation for her to have children soon had set the 'bar too high'. Tess was experiencing incongruence, which revealed itself through tears of frustration. This was a new but unpleasant experience for Tess.

By associating success with what she could achieve, Tess had ignored her real feelings and had lost the quality of experiencing the here and now. She realised that she had not enjoyed her wedding because Tess was so focused on its perfection:

*Tess*: Even my wedding had to be just so. When I look back I was bossing everyone around, stressing about the flowers and dresses and vows. It was such a massive task and I couldn't let anyone do anything in case they messed up.

*Therapist*: It was a massive task that you needed to be in control of all by yourself.

*(Continued)*

*(Continued)*

*Tess*: I was like a mad woman! And all I really wanted to do was run away to Vegas with him [*husband*] without any hassle. You know, our way, just as we wanted it?

Tess also realised that she had not travelled to places which she had imagined as a child because backpacking was seen as a 'waste of education' by her family. Her focus on being an ideal successful business woman had squashed any desires to do something she wanted to do for fun. Overall, Tess was not free just to enjoy her life as she experienced each moment. The fear of being judged or rejected by her loved ones was too overpowering. Success had become an additional load for Tess's own back rather than a positive sense of achievement or growth.

The incongruence between her real self and ideal self was causing her much confusion. Her self-concept had become torn between the two states of being: either the successful ideal self or the hidden desired self (see Figure 8.5).

Eventually, as therapy progressed, Tess began to experience her real self and trust her feelings, thoughts and reactions. She began to question what she actually wanted from her life. The realisation that having children was not something she or her husband wanted right now came as a relief. Instead, she came to understand that this was something her parents thought she ought to do.

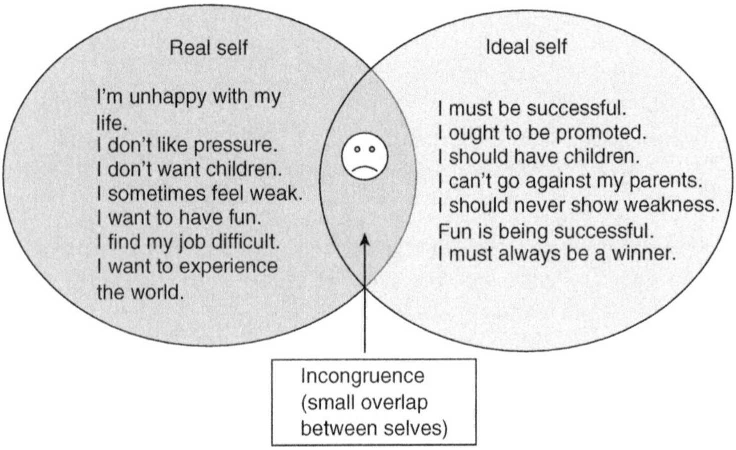


**Figure 8.5** The incongruence between Tess's real self and ideal self

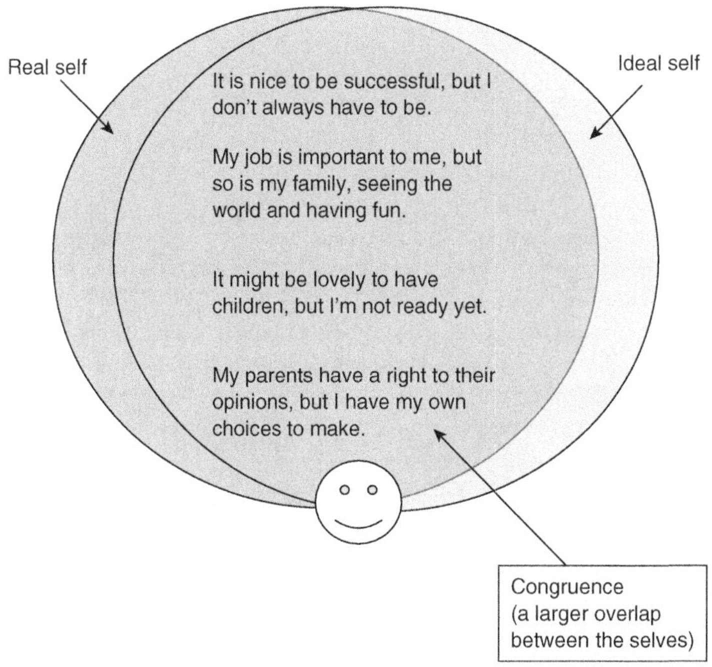


**Figure 8.6** Tess achieves congruence

Over the sessions Tess got in touch with her inner desires, feelings and deeper thoughts. She began to feel a confidence that was genuine and started to trust in her inner feelings. Rather than ignore or mask them, Tess experienced them as they happened. Tess began to trust herself and listen to what she actually wanted in life. She started to make decisions based on this without the fear of failure inhibiting her.

Although Tess was aware of some of the conditions of worth and expectations around her, she began to 'fully function' with her whole self rather than a fractured self. Tess became open to experiences that she previously ignored (e.g. planning a backpacking trip), embraced changes (deciding not to have children just yet) and put trust in her inner thoughts, feelings and behaviours. Tess began to ease the focus from achieving the ideal and instead embracing the 'real Tess' (see Figure 8.6).

By being more realistic and recognising 'who' rather than 'what' Tess wanted to be, she ended therapy in a congruent state. She was more open to her feelings and experiences, and ready to embrace changes. Tess was ready to have fun!

## HISTORY

Carl Rogers (1902–1987), the founder of PCT, was born in America and worked there throughout his life. His writings were heavily influenced by the work of Carl Jung. However, his therapeutic approach was largely based on his personal and clinical experience.

Rogers believed in a new approach to therapy which went against the prominent approaches of his time (e.g. psychodynamic psychotherapy/behaviourism). He and a few others, such as Abraham Maslow (known for the pyramid of human needs) and Clark Moustakas (known for his work on play therapy), originated the branch of psychology called 'humanistic psychology'. This approach went against the idea that human beings had little choice over their lives and were often driven by biological forces. It also went against the view that people needed an expert to tell them where they had 'gone wrong' or how to 'mend' themselves.

Rogers' 'non-directive therapy' (later known as 'client-centred' therapy) adopted the stance that the person accessing therapy would be able to find their own answers to problems. Rogers trusted that individuals would always develop towards their full potential. His approach to psychotherapy and counselling at the time (1940s–1960s) was considered revolutionary. It also received a lot of criticism because the approach emphasises personal qualities rather than techniques in therapy.

Although Rogers' approach was initially developed as an approach to psychotherapy, like-minded humanistic colleagues came to understand that it could also be transferred outside the therapeutic environment. They believed that it could be used wherever relationships were important (e.g. work, schools, patient care, childcare). Consequently, the term 'client' was replaced with 'person' to make the approach more widely applicable and accessible.

Some people find objection to the 'appropriation' of the term 'person-centred' (e.g. Mearns and Thorne, 2007: 3), the argument being that it can often be used without true grounding in PCT. Mearns and Thorne suggest that if PCT were truly and more widely adhered to, it would mean a move away from 'the target-driven, efficiency-obsessed, surveillance monitored environment prevailing in so many professional fields at this time' (2007: xiii).

In the later years of Rogers' life, he began to further develop the person-centred approach by defining the element of 'presence' required by the counsellor or facilitator role. Unfortunately, he died in California (aged 85) before completing this work. However, other writers, such as Brian Thorne or Dave Mearns, continue to expand on Rogers' ideas, and his humanistic approach continues to guide many of us in our daily lives and relationships many years after his passing.

There are still conflicting views amongst the various tribes of PCT about how the approach is developing. However, as with all evolving therapies, there will inevitably be those who could be termed 'purists' and those who have contributed to the development of the approach. If you are particularly interested in this evolution, but perhaps lean more towards the purist end of the spectrum, it would definitely be worth having a read of Mearns and Thorne's (2007) book *Person-Centred Counselling in Action*.

## GLOSSARY

| | |
|---|---|
| Conditional acceptance | Being accepted by other depending on their imposed conditions and expectations. |
| Conditional regard | Being regarded by others depending on their imposed conditions and expectations. |
| Congruence | A balanced overlap between the real self and ideal self. |
| Core conditions | The six conditions that are central to PCT. |
| Empathic understanding | Trying to understand the experience of others and how that experience may affect them. |
| Facilitation | The therapist role: to facilitate rather than lead therapy. |
| Fully-functioning person | A psychologically healthy person. |
| Ideal self | The type of person we would ideally like to be. |
| Incongruence | A lack of balanced overlap between the real self and ideal self. |
| Incongruent position | A state of instability when a person feels torn between their real self and ideal self. |
| Non-directive therapist | A therapeutic approach that uses facilitation rather than direct control. |
| Organism | The word Rogers liked to use to describe an individual. |
| Organismic valuing process | The inner process that involves our feelings, thoughts and reactions upon which we base our likes, dislikes, safety and experiences. |
| Real self | The true and actual person we are. |
| Reflection | A therapeutic skill expressing the experience of a person and the therapeutic relationship at any point throughout therapy. |
| Self-actualising tendency | The innate drive to develop in the best way we can with the resources we have available (also referred to in this chapter as 'best potential'). |
| Self-concept | The perception of ourselves based on our own thoughts and what we think others judge us as being. |

| | |
|---|---|
| Self-worth | How well we value ourselves. |
| Therapist's congruence | The therapist's role to be honest and genuine with themselves and the person, rather than being disingenuous, the expert or leader. |
| Unconditional acceptance | Receiving acceptance from others for all that you are without conditions applied. |
| Unconditional approval | Receiving approval or love from others whatever you do unconditionally. |
| Unconditional positive regard | Being well regarded by others without imposed conditions. |

## REFERENCES


Casemore, R. (2006) *Person-Centred Counselling in a Nutshell*. London: Sage.

Mearns, D. (1994) (ed.),'Don't confuse unconditional positive regard with 'liking', in D. Mearns, *Developing Person-centred Counselling*. (pp. 3-4). London: Sage.

Mearns, D. and Thorne, B. (1988) *Person-centered Counselling in Action*. London: Sage.

Mearns, D. and Thorne, B. (2007) *Person-centered Counselling in Action* (3rd edn). London: Sage.

Rogers, C. R. (1951) *Client-centred Therapy: Its Current Practice, Implications and Theory*. London: Constable.

Rogers, C. R. (1959) 'A theory of therapy, personality and interpersonal relationships as developed in the clients centre framework', in S. Koch (ed.), *Psychology: A Study of Science, Volume 3: Formulations of the Person and the Social Context* (pp. 184-256). New York: McGraw Hill.

Rogers, C.R. (1961) *On Becoming a Person: A Therapist's View of Psychotherapy*. London: Constable.

Saunders, P. (2006) *The Person-centered Primer: A Concise, Accessible Comprehensive Introduction*. A Steps in Counselling supplement. Ross-on-Wye: PCCS Books.

Tolan, J. (2003) Skills in *Person-centered Counselling and Psychotherapy*. London: Sage.

## Worksheet 8.1

# The techniques of reflection

Typically, five main forms of reflection are used (Mearns, 1994: 122–123) by a therapist and are briefly detailed here.

1. **Situational reflection:** The therapist reflects on people, places, objects or events. This is thought to help the person connect with their present environment. For example:

   *Therapist*: It's a bit cold in here, but it should warm up soon.
   *Therapist*: The room's been moved around a little since we last met.

2. **Facial reflection:** The therapist reflects on the emotion observed on the face of the other person to help them connect to pre-expressive feelings. For example:

   *Therapist*: You look a little nervous.
   *Therapist*: You're gritting your teeth.

3. **Body reflection:** The therapist reflects on the person's posture, movements or gestures by either physically mirroring them or verbally expressing them. This aids the person's sense of body with the current moment. For example:

   *The therapist leans forward towards the person in reflection of the person's posture (non-verbal reflection) to communicate shared interest.*
   *Therapist*: You stamped your foot as you said 'no'.
   *Therapist*: You're all curled up on the seat.

4. **Word-for-word reflection:** The therapist reflects phrases, words, sentences or sounds used by the person, which seem meaningful to them. This is thought to help the person experience expressing themselves and help them familiarise themselves with this use of speech. For example:

   *Therapist*: This state of being feels 'stale' for you.
   *Therapist*: You're all 'out of sorts' … all over the place.

5. **Reiterative reflection:** Previous reflections are repeated to facilitate the contact within the therapeutic relationship and the person's connection to their present experience. For example:

   *Therapist*: I said, this state of being feels 'stale' for you and you looked at me and then at the cooling fan. Maybe it feels stale in this room too?

# Worksheet 8.2

## Incongruence in relation to difficulties

**Real self**

I'm emotionally hurt.
I'm afraid of being vulnerable.
I'm angry.
I'm ashamed of my behaviour.

**Ideal self**

I should never be vulnerable.
Others shouldn't make me angry.
I should always be in control.

**Example b) an anxious individual:**

**Real self**

I am so afraid.
I don't like certain situations.
Sometimes I frighten myself.
I have awful thoughts.

**Ideal self**

I should be confident and capable.
I should never be afraid.
I should act normal like everyone else.

**Example c) a depressed individual:**

**Real self**

I feel angry, hurt and let down.
I feel so hopeless.
I don't feel loved or lovable.

**Ideal self**

I should be happy like everyone else.
I should never get angry with others.
I ought to get over this and on with my life.

# Worksheet 8.3

## Thinking about the person in therapy

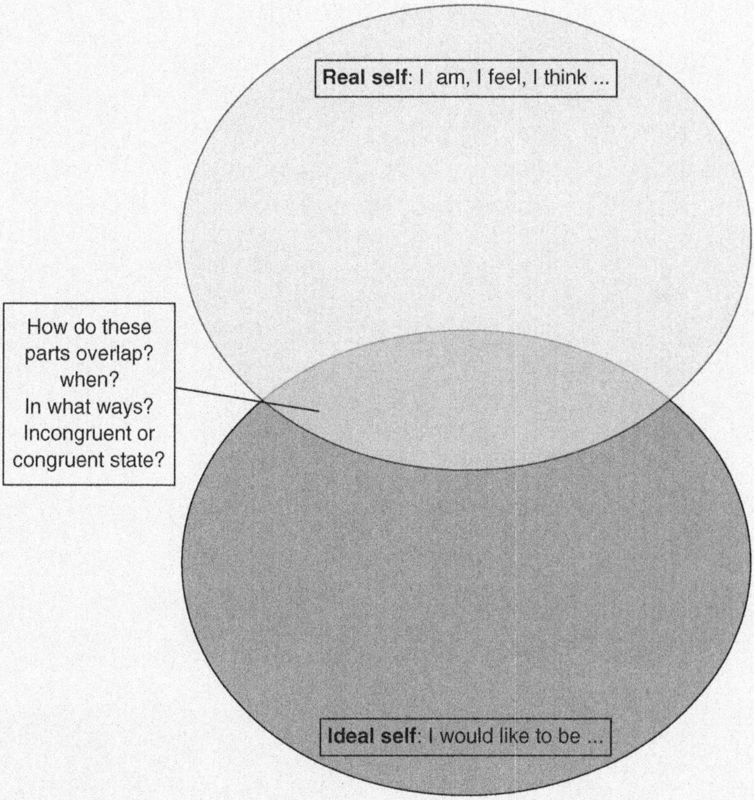


Pressures, demands or expectations I feel or have experienced:

# Worksheet 8.4

## Wearing masks

This worksheet can be used in therapy to gain an understanding of a person's perception of their ideal and real self, through the metaphor of wearing masks. Sometimes we try to cover up our true feelings by presenting what we think other people want to see. You might say it's like wearing a mask to present our ideal self to the world.

### Wearing the mask

1. Have you ever worn a (metaphorical) mask to cover your true feelings? If so, when do you tend to wear the mask?

2. When wearing this mask, what do you try to portray to others? (e.g. That you were: confident, brave, clever, attractive, humble, etc)

### Behind the mask

What does the mask cover up? When you don't have the mask on, what kind of a person are you and what feelings do you have about your self?

# 9 MINDFULNESS

## Katie Splevins

Emerging from Eastern meditative traditions, mindfulness is the ability to attend to experiences in a certain way. It involves training the mind to focus attention towards internal and external events in the present moment in a kind and compassionate way. One of the many benefits of mindfulness therapy is learning to distinguish between raw experiences and the conditioned judgements and conclusions we often bring to them. By compassionately noticing and accepting thought patterns as internal events rather than 'facts', people can begin to distance themselves from unhelpful or automatic responses and be empowered to make more deliberate and helpful choices in response to life events. Although mindfulness therapies often teach mindfulness meditation as a distinct skill, benefit is greatest for those who incorporate mindfulness into their whole lives where it has the power to produce profound personal transformations.

## THE MODEL

### What is mindfulness?

Mindfulness meditation has been defined as 'paying attention in a particular way; on purpose, in the present and non-judgementally' (Kabat-Zinn, 1994: 4). It is, however, about much more than just reigning in a wandering mind. The aim is to notice what is going on in the body, the mind and indeed daily life in an accepting and non-judgemental way, hence it has been termed 'the art of conscious living' (Kabat-Zinn, 1991). This might well contrast with our more usual mode of 'automatic pilot' (e.g. driving to work and forgetting the journey).

Mindfulness meditation is based on the assumption that much suffering stems from operating unconsciously in the world. Due to this lack of awareness people may respond unquestioningly to well-trodden thought patterns, ideas and expectations, even when they are not helpful. Within a therapeutic context, a person can learn to meditate and then work together with a therapist to recognise when common but unhelpful thought patterns arise. Usual responses and actions to these thought patterns can then begin to be observed rather than responded to unconsciously.

Grounded in Eastern meditative traditions such as Hinduism, Buddhism and yoga, mindfulness meditation can be traced back more than 2,500 years. Despite originating within religious and spiritual scriptures, it is worth noting that mindfulness meditation does not require any religious affiliation; In fact, mindfulness meditation has been incorporated into various secular therapeutic approaches, often referred to as 'third-wave therapies' (see References at the end of this chapter).

The goal of mindfulness therapy is the development of 'insight'. Insight is viewed as very different to thinking; Indeed, reasoning or thinking as a way of increasing understanding is viewed as a possible contributor to difficulties, as thoughts may represent personal or social constructions of events. Instead, mindfulness meditation aims to:

- Teach people to greet experiences as if for the first time rather than anticipating predicted conclusions.
- Stay with difficult experiences rather than avoiding them.
- Train people to develop 'meta-cognitive insight' (Teasdale, 1999), which is the ability to witness thoughts, perceptions, emotional reactions and physical sensations as unbiased observers.
- Help people to live in the present moment rather than the past or future.

> Mindfulness has also been acknowledged among Western meditative tradition including Native American teachings. To find out more, read the works of Americans Walt Whitman and Henry David Thoreau.

> Meta-cognitive insight has been found to be particularly useful in relapse prevention for people with depression (Teasdale et al., 2000).

In this way people can develop insight and wisdom, which in turn allows them to become:

- Liberated from patterns of thinking and behaving that previously added to their suffering.
- Observers of their internal events, treating events as passing clouds, thus resisting the urge to engage with them or act them out.
- Aware of their likes, dislikes, desires, expectations and prejudices.
- Able to live in the present and engage with raw experiences as they arise.

In Buddhism, this wisdom is sometimes called 'enlightenment'. It shares similarities with Maslow's (1968) description of a self-actualised person, and with the positive psychology paradigm; both of which refer to the possibilities of developing positive states of mind that go beyond symptom relief. In this way, mindfulness meditation is more than just a new coping tool for a person to draw on but often becomes a way of life.

## APPLICATION

The effective application of mindfulness meditation training relies on four core components: a commitment to meditating; development of the seven pillars of mindfulness (Kabat-Zinn, 1991); connecting with present moment experiences; and therapist use of mindfulness practice.

### A commitment to meditating

The words 'mindfulness meditation' may conjure up all sorts of associations for people (including the possibility of levitation). However, it is nothing more than simply turning your awareness towards yourself, your internal events, cognitions, perceptions and desires, and beginning to see more clearly how they operate in your life. It is about bringing curiosity to ongoing internal processes rather than the content of them. Mindfulness meditations can last anything from a few minutes to retreats lasting months or years. To gain the benefits, a person needs to meditate regularly.

When setting up a formal mindfulness meditation practice there are several points to consider (discussed in detail in Worksheet 9.2). These include:

- **Meditation position**: The position should reflect a sense of alertness and commitment to being attentive, rather than promoting sleepiness.
- **The breath**: While it is not essential to meditate on the breath, it is often used during meditation practice as an 'anchor' to the present moment.
- **Types of meditation**: The ways in which a person can bring awareness to the present moment are limitless. Almost any sensory experience can be meditated on (e.g. breathing, eating, seeing, listening and body sensations).
- **Inquiry**: Following meditation, a period of time devoted to sharing experiences is often useful, particularly for beginners. The purpose of an inquiry is to encourage people to be curious about experiences that have arisen during the mediation and to become more knowledgeable about themselves.

When following a meditation with an inquiry, it is worth bearing in mind the key learning points when you explore the experience of people (see Table 9.1).

| | |
|---|---|
| 1. | Helping people to make mindful decisions at points when they have a choice. |
| 2. | Linking being mindful in formal practices with mindfulness in daily life. |
| 3. | Decentring – learning to witness thoughts and feelings rather than being them. |
| 4. | Learning to accept an experience as it is. |
| 5. | Learning to see recurring patterns in the mind and how they progress. |
| 6. | Developing a position where you can fully be with an experience and simultaneously observe it. |
| 7. | Learning to recognise the raw experience without judgement or labels. |
| 8. | Encouraging compassion towards the self and others. |
| 9. | Encouraging curiosity. |
| 10. | Using the breath as an anchor. |
| 11. | Learning how to direct attention and also disengage it. |

**Table 9.1** Key learning points to consider in meditation

## The seven pillars of mindfulness: cultivating a particular attitude

The aim of mindfulness meditation is to develop increased awareness of internal and external events. However, it is crucial that this task is approached in a non-striving and patient way with kindness, non-judgement and acceptance. The focus is on letting go of experiences, and trying to retain what is termed a 'beginner's mind', when exploring the present moment. Kabat-Zinn (1991) reflected the importance of this attitudinal stance and described them as the 'seven pillars of mindfulness', which support the efficacy of the practice. It can be useful to help people refer regularly to the seven pillars of mindfulness before and after they meditate as a way of helping them become familiar with their own ways of approaching experiences. The seven pillars are shown in Figure 9.1 and discussed below.

### 1. Non-judging

'I'm useless at this', 'This is awful', 'Meditation is ridiculous!'– these are all common examples of negative judgements related to experiences which might arise for people. Equally common are positive judgements often related to what we feel we need, want, deserve or desire. 'I shouldn't be judging myself' is just another judgement. It is not unusual to find an almost constant flow of judgements in response to our internal and external experiences that we normally fail to question.

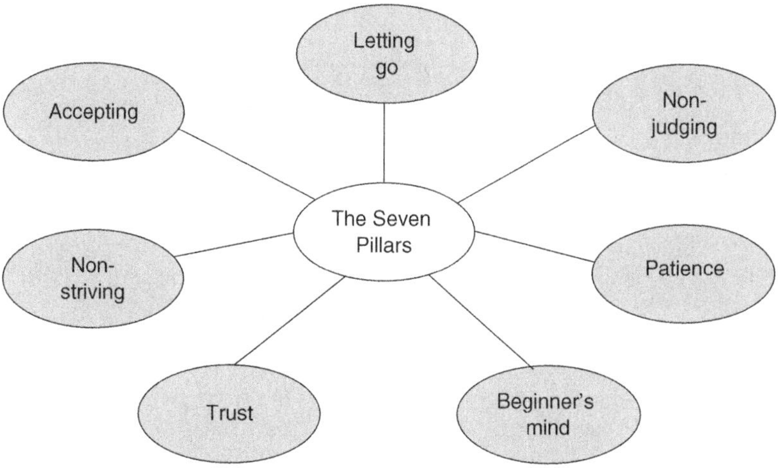


**Figure 9.1** Kabat-Zinn's seven pillars of mindfulness

This, often unconscious, habit of labeling things 'good' or 'bad', 'right' or 'wrong', may actually add to the stressors we experience in our lives. Such judgements may lead people to reject or avoid experiences or to cling to impossible dreams. Listening for judgements may also reveal a person's 'inner critic', perpetually telling them they're not good enough or are failing to achieve.

> For a great overview of the benefits of compassion and how to introduce it into your life, read Paul Gilbert's *The Compassionate Mind* (2009).

Mindfulness meditation is not about disputing an inner critic, but simply provides an opportunity to start noticing such judgements. Just by noticing them the person has a chance to see how they operate in their life and whether they add to their distress. Many people believe self-criticism is a motivating factor for self-improvement, but changes can come about more quickly when we bring compassion to our experience. Becoming aware of this also allows people to begin to behave more kindly towards themselves.

## 2. Patience

This is the ability to accept change in its own time and to allow a process to unfold without trying to rush it. In the early stages, people can notice feelings of frustration as they struggle to control the mind, and try to 'get the hang' of meditation as quickly as possible. The person may also find themselves sitting down to meditate with a plan that this meditation will 'make me better'; this is an indication of desiring immediate benefits but perhaps not putting in the practice. The same patterns can be seen in people's daily lives where they impatiently forgo the present moment and try to rush on to some imagined better future moment. As with all experiences approached mindfully, the task is simply to observe what is going on, accept this, and not let it dictate behaviour.

Patience is also considered a form of wisdom leading to 'equanimity' – a Buddhist term meaning to calmly bear difficult experiences. Equanimity is about developing a balance of mind. This is the ability to remain composed and even-minded, even when circumstances around a person appear out of control. It is facilitated by a patient and compassionate approach toward oneself and others, by which we allow events to unravel in their own way without craving for them to be different. Like a mountain enduring a storm, a person can remain steady, composed and grounded until the storm passes.

**Example:** Mohammad was a 19-year-old law student suffering from stress and anxiety related to his schoolwork and family pressures. He was becoming increasingly frustrated with himself for not seeing immediate changes in his levels of anxiety after only two therapeutic sessions, despite listening to meditation CDs two or three times a day between sessions.

Open and broad questions such as 'What did you notice about that meditation?' and 'What was interesting about that experience for you?' revealed that Mohammad experienced inpatient feelings and thoughts when he meditated. He was struck by his desire to 'get through it' and 'see results' and an anxiety that he would 'fail'. By inquiring about Mohammad's experience of impatience with the meditation, he began to notice that impatience played a key part in much of his life. For example, he approached his schoolwork in a similar way, wanting immediate results and attempting to complete assignments far earlier than his peers in order to manage his anxiety. This placed extra pressure on him, which led to increased anxiety and unnecessary stress. Furthermore, Mohammad noticed that by always impatiently rushing towards the next moment, he ended up missing out on most of his here and now.

Mohammad began to practice noticing impatient feelings arise during his meditation practice and was able to hold this in his awareness without feeling rushed. Mohammad reported finding his meditations much more enjoyable and his anxiety to lessen. Over time Mohammad began to apply this approach towards impatience in other areas of his life, allowing him to resist the urge to complete assignments in record time and thus dramatically reducing the stress he experienced in relation to his schoolwork.

### 3. Beginner's mind

In mindfulness meditation we greet all experiences with a beginner's mind. This allows us to discover a world of experiences, normally taken for granted

Cultivating a 'beginner's mind' is about trying to approach even familiar experiences as if for the first time, without predictions of what something will be like. Ordinarily we fail to really bring curiosity to many of our familiar experiences, relying on prior conditioning to tell us whether we like or dislike them and then wanting or avoiding them accordingly.

This way of thinking can be brought to a person's awareness by choosing a familiar object, for example a strawberry, and asking the person to imagine they had never seen such a thing before. The therapist can then guide the person to use their senses to really explore the strawberry. A person may find themselves in awe by the complexity of the fruit, or if it is a fruit they dislike they might find themselves approaching it with disgust.

Whatever the experience, it provides an opportunity for a person to see how rarely we approach something with a neutral mind, and people are usually surprised at how little they have noticed the smell, taste, texture and look of such a common fruit. Even taking a breath, hardly a new experience for any of us, can be approached with a beginner's mind. After all, no two breaths are exactly the same, and no breath has ever before been experienced in *this* moment. However, we usually only examine things that are new and generally imagined as positive.

### 4. Trust

We are often advised to ask others – experts, teachers, parents – for their opinion on what to do in difficult situations, and many of us rely on such tutors for knowledge throughout our lives. While advice from others can be valuable, it needs to be sought without neglecting one's own inner wisdom. Ultimately, people know themselves and their needs more intimately than anyone else. Mindfulness meditation provides a vehicle to become reacquainted with this often neglected inner voice.

**Example:** Jack, a 46-year-old male, had suffered for several years with pain related to fibromyalgia. He had previously been a fit and active man but was finding his gym regime and working hours were too much for him and worsened the pain. Jack's wife felt that Jack needed to push himself and not 'give in' to the pain. Jack felt he was letting his family down and felt unable to improve his situation as the pain worsened. He was becoming irritable and snappy with his family, which increased his sense of being useless and lowered his mood.

Jack began a yoga class, initially as a gentle form of exercise but also as a way of practising mindfulness meditation through movement. Jack discovered that when he paid attention to his body it was clear when he was overstraining and pushing himself. He also noticed that he often disregarded his own intuition telling him when he needed to stop, in favour of his wife's words to not 'give in'. With practice, Jack began to trust this inner voice and take responsibility for adapting the exercises to suit his ability without comparing himself to the ability of others. He found that by exercising moderately and in tune with his body, he was able to gain some physical exercise but not agitate his condition. Jack's mood improved, as did his family relationships.

## 5. Non-striving

The idea of undertaking a task without striving for a particular end point is an alien concept in much of Western culture. Mostly we aim to achieve something or 'get' somewhere. This has been described as the 'doing mode', which is future-focused and can limit a person's ability to attend to the present. In contrast, mindfulness meditation is about experiencing the world through the 'being mode' – that is simply staying still and being with whatever arises.

> Non-striving is not the same as doing nothing, and once a person stops expecting or demanding results they might find that results are more likely to happen.

Kabat-Zinn (1994) describes mindfulness mediation as being as much about the journey as the destination. He argues that it is the only intentional, systematic human activity which is fundamentally not about trying to improve yourself or get anywhere else, but is simply about realising where you already are.

**Example:** Lily was a 83-year-old woman who had experienced acute stomach pain for two years. Despite countless investigations there appeared to be no organic explanation for the pain. Lily was referred with depression related to the pain, which she described as constant, extreme and stopped her going out. She was no longer able to meet with her friends as she didn't want to bore them by 'moaning', so she was becoming more isolated in her home, and more focused on her pain. Lily wanted rid of the pain so she could have her life back.

Through mindfulness meditation Lily came to recognise that everything she was doing had the same end point in mind: to get rid of her pain. A failure to do so was accompanied by a series of thoughts related to a hopeless, miserable and isolated future. At the end of each meditation she would report that her pain was still present. When out with friends she would constantly monitor how bad the pain was and how it stopped her from enjoying herself. Lily was encouraged to start each sitting by just noticing her desires and striving, but not clinging to them.

By practising mindfulness, Lily became very familiar with these thought patterns and was able to distance herself from them. She found that her goal to rid herself of pain was stopping her living her life in the here and now. Over time Lily stopped striving to be without the pain and focused on her moment-to-moment experiences. She found that, in fact, the pain was not as constant as she had thought. Furthermore, at times when she was able to just 'be' with the pain as a 'sensation' to be noticed rather than responding to her associated negative thoughts about how it would spoil her fun, Lily was able to take up some of her hobbies and friendships again which brought her a great deal of pleasure.

## 6. Accepting

This refers to accepting the reality of the current experience *as it is*. If we are in pain or feel sad, then this is how it is for us at that moment. Often by trying to avoid difficult emotions, sensations or feelings, or attempting to change the situation, we end up adding to the suffering. Like Lily in the above example, mindfulness meditation can help people learn to accept or even welcome difficult thoughts, sensations and emotions. Rather than fleeing from them or using avoidant or self-destructive coping strategies, people can come to realise the experience is more tolerable than they anticipated. By accepting emotionally intense experiences, rather than being carried away by them or suppressing them, people can see they are nothing more than a fleeting, transient experience.

A really nice analogy to use with clients is that of being stuck in quicksand. The more you try to get out of the situation, avoid being stuck and escape, the deeper you sink. Actually accepting that you are stuck (although not ideal) and seeing the situation as it is, is a much better first step to finding a way out.

Adopting an accepting stance is not the same as being passive. Acceptance is not about giving up or feeling helpless, or people accepting the way they cope with things. In fact, it's just the opposite; by accepting the present experience without getting tangled up in reactions and automatic responses, people can be empowered to make clearer choices about how they respond in the next moment and do what is right for them.

## 7. Letting go

The mind has a habit of attaching itself to certain ideas, hopes, fantasies, self-identity and situations. Usually we cling to those we like the sound of, and try to get rid of those we think of as unpleasant. This doesn't seem to actually make one or another experience more or less likely, it just adds another layer of distress (i.e. not being able to control our situation). By letting go of expectations and a desire for things to be a certain way, the person is liberated from self-imposed suffering and can just be with things as they are.

This can be experienced in the therapy room with something as simple as a ticking clock. When meditating, people can find this noise intensely annoying and claim it ruins their meditation and the clock needs to be removed. In fact, such a response provides the therapist with a perfect opportunity to draw attention to our desire to have experiences occur a certain way. Meditation actually can be done anywhere, anytime, and by noticing our responses to events or noises which 'interrupt' our meditation, we can see on a tiny scale how they have potential to add to our own distress and alter the course of our actions.

## Connecting with present moment experiences

The third key element related to the application of mindfulness relates to present moment awareness. Once a person begins to attend to the here and now, they begin to notice how much time is spent absorbed in past memories, future plans or worries. When in a state of mindfulness, a person has a chance to reconnect with the present moment and relieve themselves from continual imaginings and ruminations.

Although formal meditation techniques provide opportunities to place oneself in the present, informal meditative techniques often complement this process. Informal meditations can be something as simple as noticing how it feels to brush your teeth, or doing the housework in a very mindful way. It is a matter of using the everyday, the mundane, on which to meditate whenever the opportunity arises. These little spaces throughout the day give us a chance to step out of 'automatic pilot' and spend a moment or two really experiencing our lives. By focussing attention to birdsong or the sensation of a light breeze on your face, the present moment is not only pleasant but captivating.

> The three-minute breathing space is a very brief informal meditation. It can be used at any time during moments of stress or pressure, to assess what is going on for a person and to ground ourselves safely in the moment. See Williams et al. (2007).

## Therapists' use of mindfulness practice

There is currently no legal or professional requirement for those teaching mindfulness in a therapeutic context to practice mindfulness themselves. However, it has been argued that personal practice is an essential part of being an effective mindfulness practitioner, and therapists need to have their own well-established mindfulness practice in order to be effective mindfulness trainers (Segal et al., 2002: 83–84). Because of the experiential nature of mindfulness, without personal experience of the challenges, difficulties and benefits, it is very difficult for practitioners to lead appropriate inquiries or engage in discussion about what arises for people without their own experiences on which to draw. Mindfulness training courses, retreats, yoga classes, meditation groups and Buddhist centres are just a few of the places where therapists can explore their own mindfulness practice.

To conclude, mindfulness meditation is both a vehicle and an end point, allowing people the opportunity to begin to pay kindly and non-judgemental attention to what normally unfolds unconsciously, and offering an alternative to living life on 'automatic pilot'. Unlike cognitive therapy, where the emphasis is on *changing* cognitions that are considered dysfunctional, mindfulness meditation focuses on *changing our relationship with* cognitions and other internal events to one of acceptance and letting go. This ability to distance the self from thought processes is considered to be one of the mechanisms contributing to the efficacy of mindfulness. In addition, by encouraging a person to observe and explore their experiences, mindfulness can work in a similar way to exposure therapy. People are encouraged to notice any tendencies to cling to 'pleasant' experiences or avoid 'unpleasant' experiences and to try to bring a friendly curiosity to the sensations rather than fleeing. When a person meets with a raw experience, as it is, stripped from socially constructed thoughts, anticipations, judgements and reactions, they can learn to experience negative emotions and distress without coping in a self-destructive way.

## CASE STUDY

Sasha, 31, was referred by her GP for help in managing her difficulties related to eating. Sasha had carried a diagnosis of anorexia nervosa since the age of 13, but had recently lost a dangerous amount of weight following the loss of her job three months earlier. Her job loss came as a result of a mistake she had made at work for which she felt very responsible, and had triggered a sense of being useless in Sasha. Sasha had lived alone since she left home aged 17. During the initial assessment Sasha described her history to date:

Sasha had been the only girl among four brothers. Her early memories were dominated by a physically abusive and neglectful father who ruled the family home. Sasha had been very afraid of her father and felt responsible for everything that went wrong in the family home,

*(Continued)*

*(Continued)*

particularly as her father made it clear he considered her a 'mistake' and made her feel repulsive for being slightly overweight, calling her 'fatty'. Sasha's mother had been depressed for as long as Sasha could recall, and while she did try to defend Sasha at times, it usually resulted in violent arguments between her parents during which her mother got hurt. Sasha tried to cope by being 'good' at school and got good grades; however, she struggled to make friends and was badly bullied. When she was nine, Sasha started to cut herself; however, she didn't like the marks on her legs and so stopped. By the age of 13 Sasha started to purge following meals, and found this provided her with a sense of relief from difficult feelings.

As Sasha continued to describe her life story it became clear that her difficulties were being maintained in several ways:

1. Sasha had not had the opportunity to learn to emotionally regulate herself nor express her feelings as a child for fear of upsetting or angering her parents. For Sasha, feelings were viewed as something to be feared and avoided as potentially overwhelming.
2. Sasha had developed a very self-critical inner voice which she felt was useful in spurring her on to achieve at school, but which also fed into her low self-esteem, maintaining a sense that she was a 'lost cause'.
3. Sasha's coping strategy of restricting gave her a sense of control over an otherwise unpredictable life and was understood as a way of punishing herself for causing her mother so much misery. The weight loss which ensued, however, initially attracted compliments from people at school which motivated her to continue.

Before long Sasha felt she was unable to break the cycle, and the urge to purge following meals was too much to resist, as was the urge to exercise. Sasha found herself withdrawing from social life as her time was taken up constantly ruminating and planning how she would manage her next meal-and-purge cycle, leaving little time in her life for anything else.

Sasha's reasons for seeking therapy were: to find ways of coping that didn't involve food; to put on weight; and have a 'normal' life. To help achieve these goals, Sasha was initially given some reading materials introducing her to mindfulness. Sasha reflected on these in session, and stated that she had 'missed out' on her life so far and wanted to re-gain as much of it as possible. At this point we introduced a 'beginner's mind' meditation exercise, using the exploration of a raisin as a focus point (Kabat-Zinn, 1991). This confirmed to Sasha how much of life passed her by while she was ruminating about her eating rituals. The meditation exercise also triggered many of Sasha's cognitions about food, for example 'I will weigh more if I eat it', 'I will break my diet rules for the day and let myself down', 'I will look fatter' and 'I won't be able to cope with my emotions'. Following this exercise, the inquiry process provided Sasha with a first glimpse into how constant and influential these thoughts were.

Sasha was also introduced to a sitting meditation task, which was used in session and practised daily. This gave Sasha an opportunity to train her attention to the present moment, and to become increasingly familiar with her thought patterns. Sasha found she was rarely in the present but was very self-critical, and approached each meditation as a task to be competed 100% perfectly. Gradually, Sasha was able to notice the self-criticisms and judgements as aspects of meditation and daily life, and as maintaining elements to the eating disorder. By noticing these criticisms as an observer, without engaging in them, Sasha was able to feel some compassion for herself and more able to meditate alongside these judgements rather than according to them. Skills developed through formal meditations, such as decentring herself from thoughts, staying in the present and noticing her unique thought patterns, were further developed as Sasha used informal meditation practices. For example, Sasha picked two daily activities (tooth-brushing and walking to the bus stop), which she did as mindfully as possible.

During sessions, Sasha reported that focusing on the breath in the present moment gave her some relief; however, the remainder of the time Sasha found her consciousness dominated by thoughts and consequences of eating. Rather than fighting with these thoughts, the therapist asked Sasha whether they could be allowed to come and go. These thought patterns were likened to a default CD Sasha played regularly; however, she could turn the volume down any time and allow the CD to play in the background without having to sing along to it. Similarly, these thoughts about eating were default thought patterns which had been established over the years, but Sasha could allow them to be there and let them go without engaging in them or acting as if they were 'facts'. This enabled Sasha to make decisions about her eating and have opposing thoughts.

Later, a meditation exercise using the body and physical sensations as a focus was introduced, during which Sasha found herself regularly falling asleep. Sasha felt this was an avoidance strategy, as she didn't feel able to cope with exploring her body and associated thoughts related to

*(Continued)*

*(Continued)*

being useless and to blame. There thoughts elicited strong emotional reactions. Sasha worked on letting these thoughts be present without dominating her experience. In addition, Sasha was encouraged to meet these emotions with a 'beginner's mind', where, rather than predicting them to be overwhelming, Sasha simply described them as they arose, as if a child encountering them for the first time. Sasha found emotions of sadness, anger and shame to be present. At times when she could not stay and watch these emotions, she used her breath to ground her in the present moment. Sometimes this was painful, but Sasha found she could tolerate the emotions. Themes that began to emerge at this stage and which were a focus for ongoing work included:

- The value of staying in the present moment using mindfulness practice.
- Learning to direct attention and disengage it.
- The importance of not pre-judging experiences and developing a 'beginner's mind'.
- Staying with difficult feelings.
- Recognising familiar thought patterns but not treating them as 'facts'.
- Learning to accept experiences as they were.
- Encouraging self-compassion and kindness.
- Decentring; learning to witness thoughts and feelings rather than being with them.
- Helping Sasha to make mindful decisions at a point when she had a choice.

These themes continued to be built upon, using a range of meditations, and Sasha began to loosen her identification with thoughts about eating. This allowed her to make mindful choices, which lead her in the direction of her valued goals. Sasha slowly began to gain weight and participate in social activities without them being dominated by her eating rituals and thoughts. Sasha also discovered that she did not need to avoid her feelings and that they were more manageable than she had believed. Sasha discovered she had alternative coping strategies other than restricting, for example, staying with her thoughts and feelings, allowing them to subside, or using the breath as a refuge in the present moment. Sasha also began to use informal meditations as a way to remind her of her alternative choices in life. Sasha became kinder towards herself, allowing meditations to be whatever they were that day, rather than 'not good enough'. Similarly, Sasha was able to meet with the experiences of each day as they arose and to have compassion for herself on days when she did not manage to be as mindful as she would have liked. Over time Sasha gained weight, found another job and started to have the 'normal' life she had hoped for, but with the addition of a new mindful approach (see Figure 9.2).

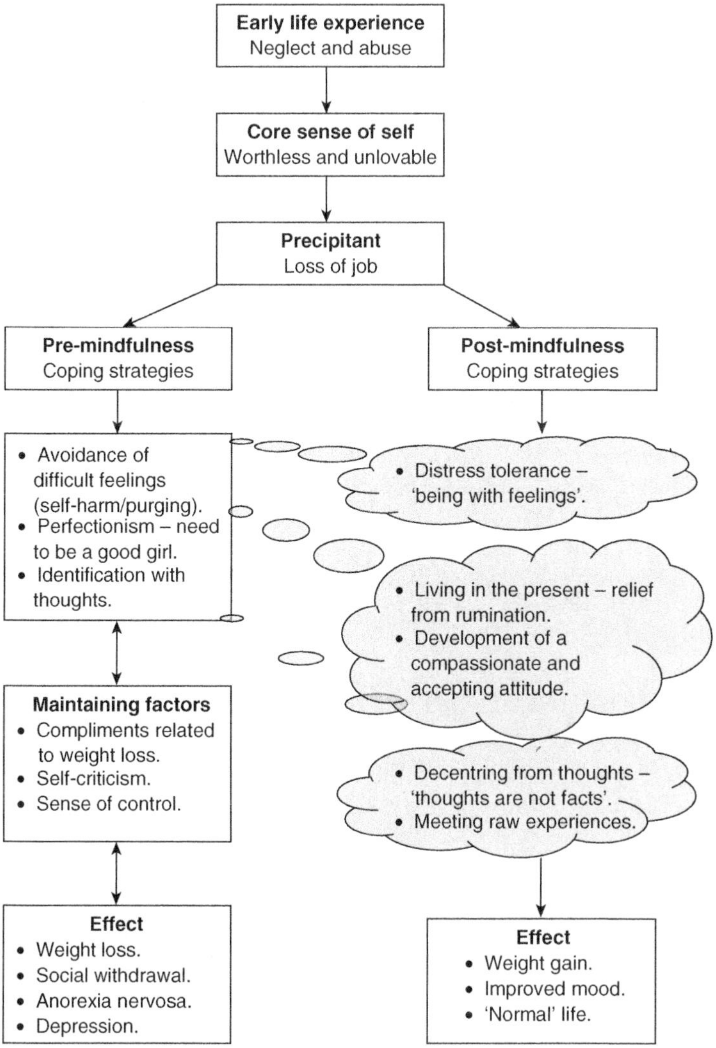


**Figure 9.2** Diagrammatic formulation utilising a mindfulness approach

## GLOSSARY

| | |
|---|---|
| Beginner's mind | Attempting to greet a new experience or sensation as if encountered for the first time, with open curiosity and a lack of judgement or expectation. |
| Being mode | Being with whatever arises in each unfolding moment without attempting to change it. |
| Compassionate mind | A way of thinking that encourages a person to recognise and tend to their own needs with warmth and understanding. |
| Conditioning | A form of learning whereby the social environment influences the development of a person's sense of self and sense of others, which they use as a template to guide their operation in the world. |
| Doing mode | A future-focused state of being where the aim is to achieve something or 'get' somewhere. |
| Equanimity | Inner balance, or the ability to remain centred regardless of difficult experiences occurring in your inner or outer world. |
| Inquiry | A period of discussion following a meditation allowing time to reflect on experiences during the meditation and increasing a person's self-knowledge. |
| Meta-cognitive insight | The ability to notice thought patterns and associated emotional responses from the position of a non-judgemental witness or observer, rather than identifying with them. |
| Mindfulness meditation | A way of directing attention, on purpose, in the present and non-judgementally, with the aim of gaining insight and alleviating suffering. |
| Observer stance | A way of viewing internal sensations and cognitions with meta-cognitive insight. |
| Seven pillars of mindfulness | Seven attitudes which support the development of insight gained by mindfulness meditation. |
| T'ai chi | A Chinese form of meditation through movement, often based on martial arts. |
| Third-wave therapy | A therapy where the focus is on relationships, personal values, mindfulness and spirituality, with an emphasis on accepting rather than trying to change things. |

## REFERENCES

*Gilbert, P. (2009) *The Compassionate Mind*. London: Constable.

*Hayes, S. C., Strosahl, K. and Wilson, K. (2003) *Acceptance and Commitment Therapy: An Experiential Approach to Behavior Change*. New York: Guilford Press.

Kabat-Zinn, J. (1991) *Full Catastrophe Living: Using the Wisdom of Your Body and Mind to Face Stress, Pain, and Illness*. New York: Delta Trade.

Kabat-Zinn, J. (1994) *Wherever You Go, There You Are: Mindfulness Meditation in Everyday Life*. New York: Hyperion.

*Lineham, M. M. (1993) *Cognitive-behavioral Treatment of Borderline Personality Disorder*. New York: Guilford Press.

Maslow, A.H. (1968) *Toward a Psychology of Being* (2nd edn). New York: Van Nostrand.

Segal, Z., Teasdale, J. and Williams, M. (2002) *Mindfulness-based Cognitive Therapy for Depression*. New York: Guilford Press.

Teasdale, J. D. (1999) 'Emotional processing: Three modes of mind and the prevention of relapse in depression', *Behavior Research and Therapy*, *37*, 53–77.

Teasdale, J. D., Segal, Z. V., Williams, J. M. G., Ridgeway, V. A., Soulsby, J. M. and Lau, M. A. (2000) 'Prevention of relapse-recurrence in major depression by mindfulness-based cognitive therapy', *Journal of Consulting and Clinical Psychology*, *68*, 615–623.

Thoreau, H.D. (1960) *A Writer's Journal* (edited by Carl Bode). New York: Dover.

Whitman, W. (1986) *Leaves of Grass*. New York: Penguin. Ebook http//:guttenberg.org/files/1322-h/1322-h.htm

Williams, M. Teasdale, J. and Kabat-Zinn, J. (2007). *The Mindful Way Through Depression*. London: Guilford Press.

## ONLINE RESOURCES AND TRANING INFORMATION

The Centre for Mindfulness Research and Practice (CMRP): www.bangor.ac.uk/mindfulness/

*Denotes third-wave therapy references

## Worksheet 9.1

## Breathing meditation

This worksheet leads you through the experience of a breathing meditation. It is not intended for use with people but as an opportunity for therapists new to meditation to become curious about their own meditative journey. The length of time you spend meditating is up to you, but 20 minutes is a good starting point. Try doing this meditation every day for a few weeks and make a note of anything that catches your curiosity or attention.

1. Find a position which is comfortable for you – possibly sitting on a straight-backed chair with your feet flat on the floor and legs uncrossed, or if you prefer, cross-legged on the floor, but make sure it is a position which you will be able to sustain comfortably for 20 minutes.
2. Sit with your back straight and your spine self-supporting. If you feel comfortable doing so, gently close the eyes. If you are not comfortable doing this, then soft-focus the eyes on a space a few feet in front of you.
3. Bring your attention and awareness to your physical presence in the room, here and now. To the space around you, the points where your body makes contact with the floor or chair, and any sensations of clothing touching the body. Spend a moment or two noticing these sensations and grounding yourself.
4. Now refocus your awareness more narrowly, to the breath. Notice the breath where it most grabs your attention. This might be as cool air coming into the nostrils, as the rise and fall of the abdomen or the movement of the chest and shoulders.
5. Spend some time following the breath with your attention. Bring a beginner's mind to the task, for each breath is unique. As best you can, follow the changing physical sensations as the breath enters and leaves the body, perhaps noticing where one breath ends and another begins. You don't need to try to breathe in any special way – let the breath breathe itself – try to let go and just watch it as an unbiased observer.

6. Try to bring an attitude of acceptance and letting go to the meditation as a whole. As best you can, simply allow your experience to be your experience without needing it to be other than it is. You may also want to bear in mind the other pillars of mindfulness – compassion towards yourself, patience, non-judging and non-striving.
7. It is likely that throughout this (and every other meditation) your mind will wander from the focus of the breath to other thoughts, intentions, plans, daydreams, worries. This is normal – it's simply what minds do – it is not a sign of failure. Once you notice this has happened gently escort your attention back to the breath and congratulate yourself on having returned to the present. You might want to briefly note where the mind has been without becoming engaged in related thoughts.
8. Keep repeating this pattern as many (million) times as you need to, Noticing that your awareness has strayed from the breath and in a kindly way, without criticism, returning the attention to your breathing.
9. Continue with the practice for 20 minutes if this feels right for you. Try to bring a sense of kindliness to the whole experience and a sense of curiosity. The aim is nothing more than to simply be aware of your present experience in each moment as best you can.

# Worksheet 9.2

## Setting up a formal meditation

| | |
|---|---|
| **Meditation position**<br>The position should reflect a sense of alertness and commitment to being attentive, rather than promoting sleepiness. | • Traditionally, formal meditation is usually undertaken in a seated position with the legs crossed and cushions to support the buttocks and knees.<br>• Other positions, such as sitting on a chair or lying down, can be used just as effectively. |
| **The breath**<br>The breath is often used during meditation practice as an 'anchor' to the present moment. | • Focusing attention on the breath provides a chance for the mind to calm.<br>• The nature of the breath (fast, slow, shallow, constricted) can provide a window into your state of mind.<br>• It may be that a whole meditation is dedicated to paying attention exclusively to the breath, or it may simply be used as an 'anchor' to the present moment if overwhelmed by thoughts or emotions. |
| **Types of meditation**<br>Ways in which to bring awareness to the present moment are limitless.<br>You can meditate on almost any sensory experience, e.g. breathing, eating, seeing, listening and body sensations. | • Mindfulness meditations can include: sitting or lying down, or activities such as walking, yoga, T'ai chi, etc.<br>• Deciding which meditation to use is partly reliant on an individual's preference.<br>• There is also an element of choosing meditations that gradually build up understanding and competence.<br>• A body-scan meditation, which encourages people to simply notice body sensations and any related feelings or cognitions, can be a good starting point (Kabat-Zinn, 1994).<br>• Meditations can be recorded onto CDs and given to people to practice at home in between sessions. |

| | |
|---|---|
| **Inquiry**<br>Following meditation, a period of time devoted to sharing experiences is often useful, particularly for beginners.<br>The purpose of an inquiry is to encourage people to be curious about experiences that have arisen during mediation and to become more knowledgeable about themselves. | • Sharing experiences about the meditation:<br>o normalises experiences, such as how often the mind wanders.<br>o provides an opportunity for therapists to help people connect their experiences with important learning points.<br>• Discussion may revolve around where sensations are physically located in their body, how internal experiences may emerge and change over time, and what reactions they had to any such experiences.<br>• It is also a chance to develop the seven pillars of mindfulness (see Worksheet 9.3).<br>• Over time people can begin to make links between the patterns that emerge during meditation sessions and their broader life experiences. |

# Worksheet 9.3

## The seven pillars

This worksheet can serve as a guide for therapists wishing to explore their own meditation experiences or those of others. The questions, based on the seven pillars of mindfulness, are examples to be used in a gentle, non-striving way.

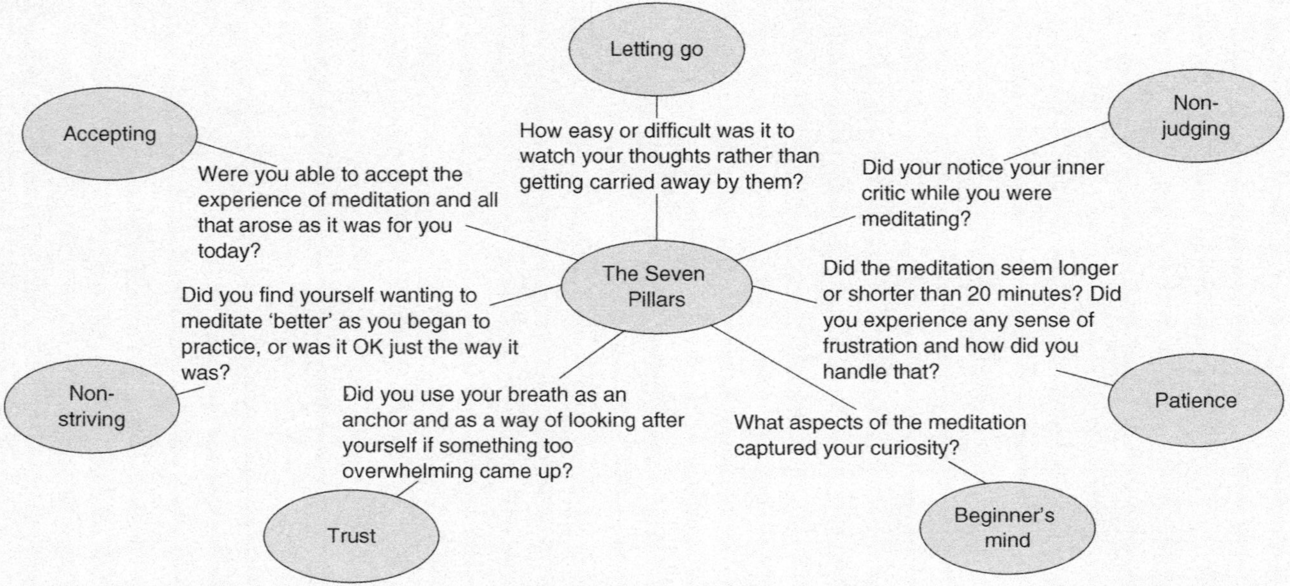

## Worksheet 9.4

## Commitment to meditation

Developing one's own commitment to meditation is considered necessary in becoming an effective mindfulness trainer. The record chart below can be used to help therapists develop their own mindfulness practice.

| Day/time spent | Meditation | Inquiry |
|---|---|---|
| Example (10 minutes) | **What did the meditation involve?** [e.g. I used the eating of a clementine as a mindfulness exercise.] | **What experiences arose during the exercise?** [e.g. At the start I noticed my mind wandering to thoughts of whether I was doing it right, I noticed this and used the breath to refocus my mind on the present moment.] |
| **Monday** Time spent: | | |
| **Tuesday** Time spent: | | |
| **Wednesday** Time spent: | | |
| **Thursday** Time spent: | | |
| **Friday** Time spent: | | |
| **Saturday** Time spent: | | |
| **Sunday** Time Spent: | | |

# 10 SOLUTION-FOCUSED BRIEF THERAPY

Graeme Flaherty-Jones
and Fiona Syme

Solution-focused brief therapy (SFBT) is a future-orientated and goal-directed model of brief therapy that was developed in the early 1980s by Steve de Shazer, Insoo Kim Berg and colleagues. SFBT is often short-term but not always time-limited. In practice SFBT pays close attention to the language used in therapy to help draw out the competence, skills and personal attributes of the person to help them overcome difficulties in their life. SFBT techniques encourage the person to increase the frequency of their problem-solving behaviour at an individual and family systems level.

## THE MODEL

### What is solution-focused brief therapy?

The solution-focused brief therapy (SFBT) model arose in the 1980s from the family therapy tradition in the USA, where Steve de Shazer and his team at the Brief Family Therapy Centre in Milwaukee found that:

- People were helped by focusing on the future rather than the problem-saturated past.
- Therapy did not have to involve long analysis.

These revelations dramatically altered their practice and led them to identify a philosophical stance and a knowledge base for SFBT.

SFBT is not theory-based but was pragmatically developed and became situated within the constructionist school of therapies, which assumes that all meaning is created by individuals rather than there being an objective reality. Thus, SFBT sees the future as being 'a hopeful place where people are architects of their own destiny' (de Shazer et al.,

> To read more on the philosophical underpinnings of SFBT and the brief problem-solving model, have a look at the work of Watzlawick et al. (1974).

2007: 3). The model also values a 'not knowing' position, in which therapy is seen as an opportunity to collaboratively construct a provisional understanding of both the problem and the solution.

It's important to point out here that SFBT is not simply 'positive thinking', but rather an inherent belief that all people have personal resources that can enable them to overcome difficulties in their life. By enabling the person to feel in control, solution-focused (SFBT) therapists seek to promote a person's autonomy in finding their own solutions (be they big or small) to help facilitate change. Sharing its philosophy with humanistic theory (see Rogers, 1951) and Buddhist thought, SFBT trusts that people are doing their best most of the time. If things aren't moving in the right direction, then the therapist needs to do things differently to help engage the person in a way that best suits them.

Within SFBT change is thought to occur through the person's increased awareness of their own resources, which can be used to construct their desired future. When problems are overcome in SFBT the person should leave thinking 'I solved that', not 'my therapist solved that'. Indeed, Berg and Dolan (2001: 3) describe how the therapist 'taps on the shoulder' of the person, expanding options where they can.

Before we start to look at how to apply the SFBT model in practice, it is important to become familiar with some key principles that underpin the spirit of SFBT (see Table 10.1).

## APPLICATION

### Therapist's position during therapy

Most SFBT therapists accept that there is an inherent power imbalance in therapy. However, when practising SFBT the therapist seeks to address this power imbalance by guiding in a non-directive manner. There is no set way to 'do' SFBT, but a constantly curious stance is essential. There are a few general ways of working that can help to foster this position, as described below.

1. **You are the expert on you**: holding a belief that the person accessing therapy has locked within them the key solutions to overcome their problem. The therapist's job is to help unlock these solutions through supportive questions and reflections. To introduce this notion you may say to the person 'You know you better than anyone else in the world ...', or 'You're a bit of an expert on you, and I would like to learn from your expertise to try and find ways to overcome the problem.'
2. **Staying focused**: this can be challenging, but a key skill in SFBT is to listen carefully and remain very focused on asking solution-orientated questions. This can be challenging for the person and therapist, but it is important to promote the person to do most of the thinking about possible solutions as they will know what works best for them.

| SFBT principle | How this affects practice |
|---|---|
| If it isn't broken, don't fix it, if it works, keep doing it, and if it doesn't work, stop! | At the heart of SFBT is a desire to help people overcome problems that *they* bring to therapy, through identifying what already works and trying to promote more of it. If a solution doesn't appear to be working, it should be dropped and more suitable alternatives explored. |
| Small changes can snowball to bigger changes. | Finding small but significant points of change can help people build confidence and hope that may eventually lead to a series of more systemic change without feeling too daunted. |
| The solution is not necessarily related to the problem. | While many models of therapy explore the problem in order to find a solution, SFBT begins by eliciting descriptions of what will be different when the problem is resolved. The therapist then works backwards to find times when the solution could or does exist. |
| Solution, rather than problem-focused language. | SFBT does what it says on the tin, whereby the therapist is selectively listening for the goal in every exchange. This principle shapes the goal-orientated style of questions in therapy. |
| Therapy as a supportive event. | SFBT therapists believe change is continually occurring. The therapist's role is to support the person in beginning the change process (in therapy) while recognising that it is not the only context in which change can/continues to emerge. |
| Problem transience. | The state of problems can fluctuate and people usually experience exceptions to the problem. Once identified, these exceptions are utilised to make change. |
| People have their own resources. | The SFBT therapist works to constantly seek and recognise inner resources within the person. This then provides opportunities to compliment the client and reinforce a sense of empowerment. |

**Table 10.1** Key principles of SFBT

**Example:** An angry father describes his son's behaviour in a problem-focused narrative, and the therapist works hard to keep the narrative solution-focused: 'OK, so you sound disappointed when David does X and Y, can you try to think of a time when you have enjoyed David's company? What was that like?'

3. **Blind faith**: the SFBT therapist needs to build the confidence to work without knowing too much about the problem (not easy for therapists trained to explore the detail of problems), but again this goes back to the key assumption that therapy is a supportive event and the principle that the solution may not be directly related to the problem.

Holding these qualities in mind is important, as is the need to develop a strong therapeutic alliance through showing compassion, empathy and a genuine desire to work collaboratively with the person during therapy.

De Shazer et al. (2007) note a number of broad interventions that can be used throughout SFBT, and it may be helpful to think of these as some overarching skills that should be used to guide all actions in SFBT:

- Looking for 'exceptions' (when the problem is not around in the same way).
- Gentle nudging to do more of what is working.
- Present future-focused questioning vs. past-focused questioning.
- Questions rather than interpretations.
- 'Compliments' to the person who is trying their best to move forward.

As with all models of therapy, SFBT, has some specific techniques and interventions that are used to help the person find ways to overcome their difficulties and move towards a future that is free of the problem which brought them to therapy. These interventions are discussed below and include: pre-session change, problem-free talk, solution-focused goals, identifying a preferred future, the miracle question, building on exceptions, experiments, resource seeking, scaling questions and positive feedback.

> For a recent overview of the outcome literature in SFBT, see Gingerich and Eisengart (2000).

## SFBT techniques

### Pre-session change

Remember the term 'exceptions' we mentioned above? Well, sometimes these exceptions (when the problem has not been around in the same way) can occur before therapy begins and thus present an opportunity to begin the solution-focused approach right from the start. Encouraging the person to notice these changes can be achieved in a number of ways. The fundamental question posed to the person is 'What kind of changes have you started to notice happening since you made the decision to come to therapy?' (see Worksheet 10.1 for an example).

If the person is able to generate even the slightest hint of change, this offers an opportunity for the therapist to begin 'solution talk', focusing on the possible strengths and resources of the person that has enabled this change to take place. This can also offer an opportunity to encourage the person to paint the picture of what the future may look like if these changes were to continue. If, on the other hand, the person feels that nothing has changed, then the therapist would simply explore what would need to happen for the person to leave the session feeling that it had been useful.

**Example:** Peter (a boy in his early teens) was referred to therapy regarding low mood and low self-esteem, related to his physical disability. Following introductions, the therapist asked Peter what kind of changes he had noticed since finding out he was coming to therapy. Peter said that things were about the same, so the therapist asked 'How have you managed to stop the problem from getting worse?' Peter said that he had become quite good at 'just getting on with it'. This presented the therapist with an opportunity to continue solution-talk by enquiring how exactly Peter is able to 'just get on with things'.

## Problem-free talk

Most people first arrive in therapy with feelings of uncertainty or apprehension. To ease this tension and help to build a rapport with the person, it can be useful to engage in 'problem-free talk' around the person's interests and hobbies by asking:

- What thing do you enjoy doing more than anything else in the world?
- What sort of things do you find interesting in life?
- Have you ever had any hobbies at any stage in your life?
- Would you opt for a good movie or a good book? What are you favourite types of (books/movies)? Why?

These conversations may also reveal clues as to the person's strengths and ways in which they like to approach things in life, which can then be used to help construct solutions to the problem.

**Example:** Greg came to therapy regarding his angry outbursts. The therapist had read that this young man was very good at basketball. In the first therapy session Greg was very withdrawn and appeared disengaged. The therapist scrunched up some paper and suggested they played a game to get to know one another. They played catch, and every time the other person was able to catch the 'ball' they were allowed to ask the person a question. This fun game enabled the therapist to engage Greg in a meaningful way and enabled the therapist to find out some of the 'problem-free' aspects of Greg's life, which were used later in their work.

## Solution-focused goals

Considering the metaphor of therapy as a journey; how do we reach our destination if we don't know where we want to end up? Just as we would set a desired destination when travelling, the therapist tries to elicit solution-focused goals from the person, which can be referred to through therapy as a monitor of progress. It is important to help set realistic goals that are achievable, rather than simply being without the problem. For example, 'I want to be able to start meeting my old friends for a coffee once a week' would be far more solution-focused than 'I don't want to be depressed any more'.

Some people may find it tricky to come up with specific goals that they would like to achieve during therapy, as they feel so overwhelmed by the problem. One way to begin eliciting solution-focused goals is by encouraging the person to think of a 'preferred future', where the problem is no longer around (or around to a lesser degree). Some of the questions SFBT therapists may use to gain a sense of the person's preferred future might include:

- What would have to happen for you to consider this session/therapy/our work together as having been useful?
- What are your hopes in coming here today?
- What might life look like if the problem was no longer around?

Each of these questions may reveal things that the person hopes to achieve in therapy, which can then be framed as goals. It is important that goals are realistic and that any achievements made are clearly attributed to the person's inner resources and competencies.

### The miracle question

If the person accessing therapy has difficulty responding to initial 'preferred future questioning', 'the miracle question' serves as a tool to help the person imagine in smaller, everyday detail, what they would like their life to be like if the problem was no longer around. The miracle question was originally devised by Steve de Shazer (1988) and has now become synonymous with SFBT as a key intervention technique. It can be helpful to find your own wording of the miracle question so that you can deliver it as convincingly as possible. Below is an example of the basic components that make up the miracle question.

> **Example:** OK, I'm going to ask you what might seem like a strange question. When you leave our session today you will carry on with the rest of your day as normal and, eventually, go to bed and slowly drift off to sleep. Then in the middle of the night while you are asleep, a miracle happens and the problem we have talked about today is completely resolved. However, because you were asleep when the miracle happened, you don't realise that this miracle took place and that the problem is gone. So, when you wake up tomorrow morning, what would be the first signs you notice that make you realise the problem is no longer around anymore?

Simply reading out the miracle question is not going to bring about change for the person, but when phrased carefully and delivered with sincerity, it can serve as a tool to open up conversations about a preferred future full of potential solutions. By asking the miracle question, we are trying to encourage rich descriptions of how the person's life will be different without the problem being present.

> It is usually better to look for what would be happening, i.e. positive change rather than just the absence of the problem.

There is often a mixed response to the miracle question during therapy; some may enjoy the imagery of it, others may find it hard to imagine a preferred future that is absent of the problem. In either case, the role of the therapist is to encourage the person to consider what life would look like in more and more detail with questions such as:

- What would you be thinking and feeling?
- What kind of things would you be doing?
- What else might happen?
- How might other people know that the problem has disappeared?
- What would other people notice about you?

**Example:** Jane was referred by her GP to see her therapist for help in managing her generalised anxiety. After arriving late for the session and in much of a fluster, the therapist calmly began to prompt Jane to think about a future without the problem through posing the miracle question:

*Jane*: Humm ... I don't know really ...

*Therapist*: [*remains silent*]

*Jane*: I suppose I wouldn't have so many racing thoughts going round my head about what I have to do that day.

*Therapist*: OK, what kind of thoughts would you have?

*Jane*: I'd be thinking about what I wanted to do before work.

*Therapist*: So, how might that affect your behaviour before work?

*Jane*: I'd spend more time doing the things that make me feel a bit more relaxed.

*Therapist*: And what would that look like?

*Jane*: Well, I'd be sat in my favourite chair with enough time to enjoy a cup of tea with my husband before I dash off to work.

*Therapist*: So you would have allowed yourself some time with your husband.

*Jane*: Yes, but it would also give me some headspace to talk through and prepare what I have to do for the rest of the day.

As can be seen in the above example, Jane has already been able to provide the therapist with a small but important issue that could help reduce her anxiety, that is, creating more time with her husband to think about the day

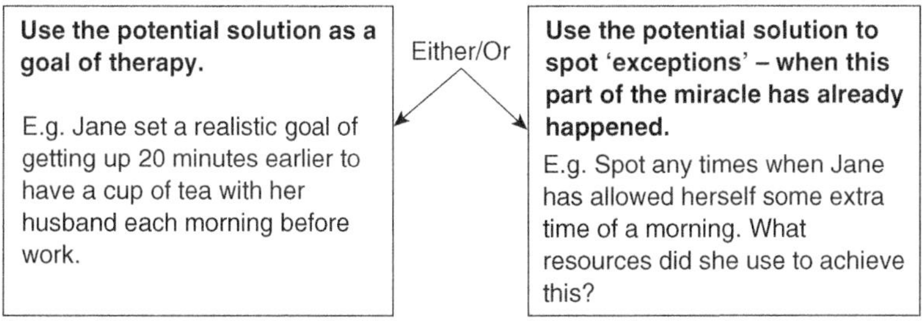


**Figure 10.1** Two ways in which Jane's potential solution can be used

ahead. When these potential solutions are discovered, they can be used in a couple of ways (see Figure 10.1).

Hopefully it is becoming clear how the miracle question can operate as a useful tool to open up conversations in which the person (knowingly or unknowingly) unveils possible solutions that can help relieve the problem. These conversations are then used to discover ways in which the solutions can be built into the person's life, and what better way of doing this than to look at times when the person has already 'done the solution' or shown 'exceptions' to the problem.

## Building on exceptions

In SFBT, 'exceptions' are considered to be times when the problem could have occurred but, for whatever reason, it did not (de Shazer et al., 2007). If the therapist wants to introduce exceptions straight after the miracle question, they may ask 'Do small pieces of this miracle ever happen, even just the slightest bit of the miracle?' If a person is able to spot a time when any aspect of their preferred future has happened, it would suggest that there has been an exception to the problem being around. This then presents the therapist with an opportunity to enquire further about this time and explore how exactly the person was able to be without the problem, which can lead to future solutions.

To follow our example of Jane, the therapist may have looked for times when Jane was able to be without the problem (anxiety) of a morning, which allowed her the precious 'thinking time with husband over a cup of tea'.

**Example:**

*Therapist*: That sounds like it would be really important to you.
*Jane*: I guess it is really, it just seems to ... you know ... calm me down a bit.
*Therapist*: Can you think of a time when this particular part of the miracle has already happened?

*Jane:* Hmm, rarely.

*Therapist:* Take a moment to think about it ... has it ever, even once, happened before?

*Jane:* Now and then on a Friday we have managed to have some brief time together.

*Therapist:* So how *did* you manage to do that?

*Jane:* Well, I just have less things to prepare that morning, so I get organised and we get some quality time before I dash off.

*Therapist:* OK, so you being organised and having things prepared seems to help?

In the above example, the therapist was able to use an exception (when the problem was not about) to highlight a potential solution (i.e. preparing things in advance can allow for quality time with husband and less anxiety) and highlight how the person's resources played a part in this exception (i.e. being organised). Whilst it can be useful to use the miracle question to find exceptions, this is not the only way to discover them.

Problems are hardly ever with people every single moment of every day. In most cases people have exceptions (no matter how brief), where the problem is not around or about in a different way. The therapist's role is to carefully and respectfully look for such exceptions and find out how, why, where and with whom they took place. It is this information that can then lead to potential solutions.

For a richer description of the differences between deliberate and spontaneous exceptions with examples, see O'Connell (1998: 61).

Exceptions can occur deliberately when the person is actively doing something they feel made a difference to the problem, or spontaneously when the problem was just not about in the same way for a reason unbeknown to the person. Spotting exceptions can be tricky, as the person may not have noticed how or why the problem was not around. It is therefore key that the therapist significantly highlights the exception, which can be done in a variety of ways:

- Repeating the exception back to the person, e.g. 'So you're saying that the depression was not around in the same way last time you visited your friend?'
- Using scaling questions to help the person explicitly rate how the exception impacted on them in that particular situation.
- Complimenting the person for their part in any exceptions, e.g. 'You should be very proud of yourself for taking the initiative to join the gym as a way to overcome the depression.'

Through marking and encouraging the person to describe the exception in rich detail, the therapist is able to gently nudge the person towards potential solutions, but fundamentally these solutions have come from the person.

## Experiments

Once an exception has been identified, the therapist should check whether this can also be transferred into a helpful solution to move the person towards their goals that were set at the beginning of therapy. A common-sense way of doing this is to try it out.

The therapist may use the term 'experiment' or 'homework assignment', but the only golden rule here is – yes you've guessed it – the experiment has to come from the person so that they have ownership. This would ideally be done by asking the person to set themselves an experiment which they feel could help. If the person is struggling, then the therapist may suggest some ideas on what the person has discussed, and below we follow on from our previous example with Jane.

**Example:**

*Therapist*: I am wondering about setting up a little experiment, but I'm not sure if you think it would be useful. How about we think a bit about your morning routine?

*Jane*: Well, I get up at 7.20 am ... I suppose I could try and get up a little earlier, hum ... say 7.00 am?

*Therapist*: Great idea, would that give you a little more time to prepare for the day and get that 'relaxed time with your husband' that you talked about?

*Jane*: Perhaps. I suppose, it's worth a shot, but I'm not sure if it'll work.

*Therapist*: Neither am I, so how are we going to know whether or not this has been successful?

Reviewing the experiment is key to finding the really helpful solutions and can often be a good way of falling back into a solution-focused conversation during the next session. A great way of reviewing experiments is through the use of scaling, as detailed below. When reviewing the experiment, any achievements or successes should be attributed to the person through identifying the resources they used to make it happen. It can also be helpful to consider the impact of the experiment on others, for example. 'What did your husband think of the experiment, did he notice anything?'

## Scaling questions

In SFBT, scaling provides a structured vehicle for asking resource, exception-seeking and preferred future questions. From the outset of therapy, scaling

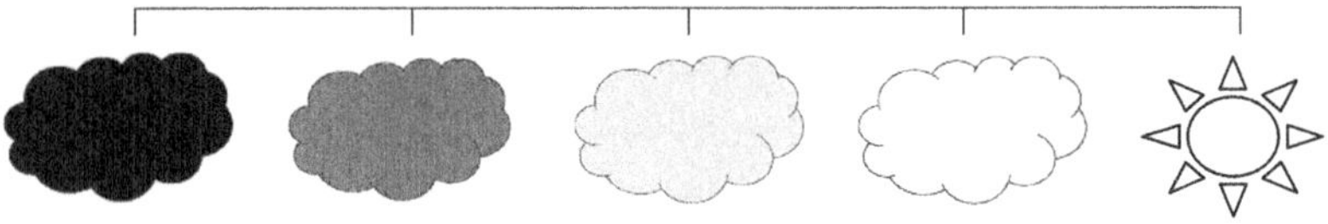


**Figure 10.2** Paul's imagery turned into a rating scale

helps to assess how much impact the problem is having on the person's life and open up conversation around what would need to happen for things to improve. Once therapy is underway, scaling can be used to measure progress, discover how motivated and confident the person is about change and to set goals. As well as using typical numerical scales (e.g. 1–10), the therapist might notice a particular metaphor that the person uses when describing the problem, which can then be transformed into a scale.

> **Example:** Paul was referred for therapy to help manage his long-standing depression. During the problem-free talk at the start of therapy, the therapist noticed that Paul frequently referred to the depression as being a dark cloud that could occasionally brighten up to be a bit patchy with a hint of sunshine. This was then used by the therapist to help construct a meaningful scale to monitor Paul's progress during therapy (see Figure 10.2).

Once the scale has been introduced (which may work best after the miracle question), the therapist can use the scale in a variety of ways:

- *Where the problem was on the scale at the point of referral and where it is now* – If the person is in any way higher on the scale, the therapist looks to see how they have managed to reach this level of improvement and praises their achievement. If it's the same, the therapist looks at how this progress has been maintained. If it has dropped, the therapist explores what would have to happen for it to go up.
- *To set the goals from therapy* – The therapist can use the scale to ask the person where things would need to be on the scale for them to feel as though therapy has been a helpful event. This number, image or word can then serve as a focus point to refer to throughout therapy to remain fixed on the person's goal and how they are going to get there (using resource questions).
- *To explore what a preferred future would look like when the person is one or more step higher on the scale* – When asking the person to describe what things would look like at one point higher on the scale, the therapist should

listen carefully and nudge towards possible solutions and opportunities for experiments.

- *To review experiments set between sessions* – By rating how the experiment impacted on the person's scale, conversation is quickly brought back to being solution-focused. If the experiment has lifted a score on the scale, the therapist can explore how the person managed to make the experiment work (i.e. what resources did they use).

Berg and Steiner (2003) provide a great selection of ideas on how to apply this with children.

Scaling questions are equally applicable with children and with adults. Designing a scale to have a 'unique' language between child and therapist can be especially fun for children and can empower them to make their own observations about feelings/behaviours, which may then lead to finding their own solutions (see also Worksheet 10.2).

### Positive feedback

At the end of each session, the SFBT therapist may choose to provide the person with concise positive feedback, based on the content of the session. When delivering feedback the therapist provides compliments on the person's achievement (no matter how big or small) and, based on what appears to be working, agrees experiments to work on before the next session.

## Being brief

The 'brief' in solution-focused brief therapy does not mean 'rushed' therapy. While de Shazer and his colleagues commented on how interventions don't always have to be long-term to obtain meaningful results for the person, it is perhaps better thought of as the 'minimum required intervention' (Myers, 2008: 39). So when the person feels they have reached a point of change during therapy that is sufficient for them to continue building on this outside of therapy, the therapist may look to bring the sessions to an end. To work around this ethos, it is once again important that both the person and the therapist are clear about the goals of therapy from the outset, so these can be held in mind when considering the point at which therapy has been helpful enough for the person.

So there you have it, a 'brief' tour of SFBT. Hopefully, in reading this chapter you can see how the therapy assists people to move towards a preferred future through establishing realistic goals and enabling the person to identify their own inner resources that can help achieve these goals. As with any model of therapy, it takes time and practice to get used to some of the language and specific techniques of the model, and the examples and following case study illustrate what this can look like in practice.

## CASE STUDY

Ann, a 62-year-old lady, was referred by a member of the mental health team for therapy regarding her recurrent bouts of depression. The referral noted that Ann had been treated for depression with medication, and while there had initially been some positive effects, these had since diminished and she had requested to speak to someone for a talking therapy.

After receiving the referral, the therapist spoke with a member of the mental health team who had been Ann's care coordinator for the last year and a half, and the following information was shared:

Ann experienced her first bout of depression shortly after retiring from work, aged 60. Ann had always enjoyed working in her local café, but felt she could no longer keep up with the role due to her arthritis. Ann's husband (Max) still worked part-time in a local car garage and contemplated giving up work to be with his wife; however, Ann insisted that he continue with this. Ann noticed that her depression was worse when Max would go to work and she felt a general sense of apathy, which resulted in her staying in the family home most of the day and led to her becoming increasingly isolated.

### Pre-session change and problem-free talk

When Ann arrived for her first session of therapy, she was very tearful and began by telling the therapist how she couldn't go on living with the depression any more. The therapist listened carefully and empathised with how upsetting this appeared to be for Ann. Ann continued, describing how the depression made her feel as though she was all alone in a dark basement and couldn't find her way out.

After Ann had explained about the depression, the therapist suggested that it might be helpful to get to know more about Ann herself, and asked if she had any hobbies or interests. Ann said that she had lost interest in most things, but that she used to like art and drawing. The therapist explored this further (using problem-free talk) and found that Ann particularly liked watercolour painting. As this conversation continued, the therapist noticed that Ann had stopped crying and appeared to be giving more eye contact in conversation.

Later in the session, following on from the problem-free talk, the therapist asked Ann what had changed since she decided to come for therapy. Ann felt that the problem was roughly the same, and so the therapist explored how Ann had prevented things from getting worse. It appeared that having something (therapy) to look forward to, provided Ann with a little hope for the future and prevented the depression from getting any worse.

### Miracle question

To try to introduce a future-orientated conversation and establish some therapeutic goals, the therapist presented the miracle question to Ann. In response to the miracle question, Ann and the therapist engaged in the follow conversation:

*Ann*: Well, I would probably notice it had gone after Max left for work.
*Therapist*: What exactly would you notice?
*Ann*: Well, I wouldn't go straight back to bed for a start.
*Therapist*: OK, you wouldn't go straight back to bed, so what would you be doing instead?
*Ann*: I'd have a shower and do a few things round the house, you know, like the odd spot of cleaning.
*Therapist*: And what would you be thinking while you were doing this?
*Ann*: I'd be thinking how good it is to have the motivation to do something again.

After continuing the conversation with prompting that encouraged Ann to describe the miracle day in as much detail as possible, the therapist asked:

*Therapist*: How might other people know the miracle had happened, say for example your next-door neighbour?
*Ann*: I don't know really, how would they know the problem had gone?
*Therapist*: Well, what might they see if they were to bump into you?
*Ann*: They may notice that I was getting out of the house for once.
*Therapist*: And where would you be going?

As Ann gave responses to the miracle question, the therapist made brief notes of the things that would be important to Ann if the problem was not around.

From these notes the therapist searched for exceptions by asking Ann if any part of the miracle had ever happened before. After thinking for some time, Ann told the therapist that the only time she

*(Continued)*

*(Continued)*

had been without the depression in the last two years was when she managed to go to a watercolour exhibition at the local art gallery. Ann explained how in doing this she had surprised herself and felt a bit brighter, but this soon passed the day after she had been.

## Goal setting and scaling

The therapist saw this as a good time to introduce scaling into the conversation and said: 'I noticed before that you described the depression making you feel like you were in a dark cellar. If we think of the bottom step of the cellar as being the point at which you came to therapy, and the top step being the best things could possibly be, where would you rate yourself today?' Ann rated herself as being on the second from bottom step out of ten on the scale, and so the therapist explored what had helped to move things upwards from the bottom step. The therapist also asked where Ann would need to be on the steps/scale for therapy to have been considered helpful, which was rated as 'six/seven'. From discussing what a sixth/seventh step would look like, Ann and the therapist agreed the following goals for therapy:

1. For Ann to be able to avoid going straight back to bed and do the odd task round the home.
2. For Ann to leave the house at least once a week on her own to do something and engage in conversation with other people.
3. For Ann to be able to go out with her husband once a week.

## Experiments

Building on the exception noted earlier, the therapist ended the session by suggesting they set an experiment. Together they agreed that Ann speak with her care coordinator about possibly looking for a painting class/group locally. This experiment didn't have to involve actually going just yet, but simply to demonstrate motivation to find one.

Ann returned to the second session having managed to complete the experiment, and so the therapist worked at complimenting Ann and finding out what inner resources she had used to achieve this. Scaling questions revealed that the experiment had helped to lift Ann's mood slightly to the third step on her scale.

Ann met with the therapist weekly for six further sessions, to discuss various expectations that had taken place over the week. The therapist remained focused on complimenting Ann on her achievements, attributed small changes to her inner resources and encouraged her to set her own experiments. By the end of their work together Ann reported her mood to have lifted to the sixth step on her scale and was now attending a weekly art class in the local community centre, as well as suggesting day trips to her husband. Ann decided that she did not require any further sessions, and so therapy came to a close with the therapist writing a letter describing all of Ann's achievements during her therapeutic journey (see Figure 10.3).

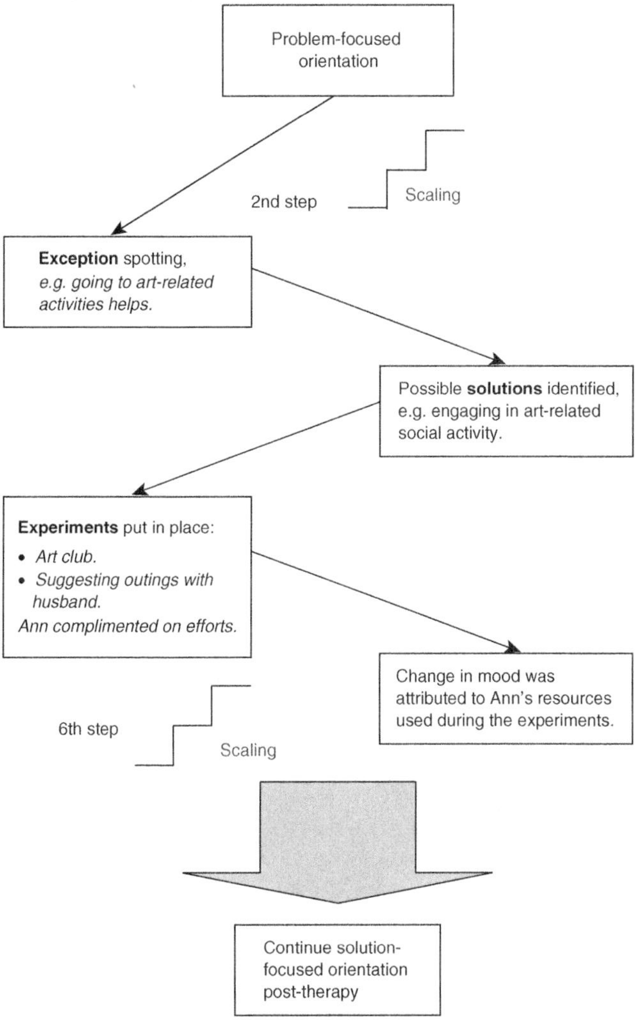


**Figure 10.3** Anne's SFBT journey

## GLOSSARY

| | |
|---|---|
| Compliments | Opportunities to compliment the person in SFBT should always be taken in line with the principle that the person should be empowered to be the 'architect of their own destiny'. |
| Competence seeking | The SFBT therapist should try to discover and reinforce the inner resources of the person, in the hope that these can be used to help solve their problem. |
| Exceptions | Times when the problem could have occurred but, for whatever reason, it did not. Exceptions present the therapist with an opportunity to enquire further about this time and explore how exactly the person was able to be without the problem, which can lead to future solutions. |
| Experiments | In SFBT, once a possible solution has been identified, the therapist should seize the opportunity to check whether or not this is a helpful solution for the person to utilise by setting up opportunities to trial the solutions out. |
| Goals for therapy | SFBT goals for therapy should be simple, clear and attainable. The SFBT therapist helps the person define very explicitly their hopes for the work in terms of understanding how the person's life would be different. |
| Miracle question | This is an intervention which is often (but not always) used in the first session to try to get the person to specify explicitly how their life would be without 'the problem'. |
| 'Not knowing' stance | The non-expert, curious stance taken by the therapist in therapy. |
| Pre-session change | The exceptions/changes that can occur before therapy begins. |
| Preferred future | The aim of SFBT is constantly to work towards the person's preferred future – a 'hopeful place' where the person can shape the landscape of their futures. |
| Problem-free talk | Conversations where the therapist can find out about the person beyond the 'problem', e.g. what are the person's hobbies and passions. This information can then help inform interventions. |
| Resource seeking | Technique whereby the therapist seeks to identify the internal resources of the person and collaboratively use these to construct a preferred future. |
| Scaling questions | A structured vehicle for asking resource, exception-seeking and preferred future questions. |

| | |
|---|---|
| Solution talk | Conversations that centre on a person's strengths and resiliencies, which can be utilised to overcome the problem. |

## REFERENCES

Berg, I. K. and Dolan, Y. (2001) *Tales of Solutions: A Collection of Hope-inspiring Stories*. New York: Norton.

Berg, I. K., and Steiner, T. (2003) *Children's Solution Work*. New York: Norton.

de Shazer, S. (1988) Clues: *Investigating Solutions in Brief Therapy*. New York: Norton.

de Shazer, S., Dolan, Y., Korman, H., Trepper, T., McCollum, E. and Berg, K. B. (2007) *More than Miracles: The State of the Art of Solution-focused Brief Therapy*. New York: Routledge.

Gingerich, W. and Eisengart, S. (2000) 'Solution-focused brief therapy: A review of the outcome research', *Family Process*, *39*(4), 477-498.

Myers, S. (2008) *Solution-focused Approaches*. Lyme Regis: Russell House.

O'Connell, B. (1998) *Solution-focused Therapy*. London: Sage.

Rogers, C. R. (1951) *Client-centred Therapy: Its Current Practice, Implications and Theory*. London: Constable.

Watzlawick, P., Weakland, J. and Fisch, R. (1974) *Change: Principles of Problem Formation and Problems Resolution*. New York: Norton.

## Worksheet 10.1

## Pre-session change

Making a decision to access therapy can be a bit daunting sometimes.With this in mind, it would be interesting to know what personal skills or traits have been drawn on in order to summon the courage to come to therapy.

**How did you summon the courage to come for therapy?**

What did you tell yourself? What did you feel? Did you have to contain your anxiety or apprehension? Are you proud of yourself? If so, for what exactly?

**What kind of changes have you started to notice happening since you made the decision to come to therapy?**

Have you noticed an ability to do something different that helps? Or not do something which helps? Or by telling yourself something it can help?

**What might the future look like if these changes were to continue?**

What might be different? For: You? Your life? Others you care about? How others treat you?

# Worksheet 10.2

## Scaling ideas

When using scaling techniques, let your creative juices run wild. The key is that it should mean something to the person (i.e. where possible use their language and things that interest them). Here are some key tips to guide you when scaling problems and therapy goals.

**Scaling problems:**

When constructing the scale remember:

- How did the person describe the problem?
- Did they use a metaphor?
- Find a way to scale its intensity which may involve: weight, intensity, severity, how often it was about, the size of the problem.

Now map this information to the scale below.

**Scaling therapy goals:**

When constructing the scale remember:

- Where did the person want to be at the end of therapy and what did they want to be happening (this is a goal)?
- How might this goal be broken up into measurable steps (e.g. distance to goal, how often the goal is already happening, percentage of the goal that has been achieved)?

Again, map this information to the scale below.

### Helpful questions to ask:

Where are you on this scale today?

*If higher than in previous session*: What has happened to allow this change to take place?

*If the same as previous session*: How have you prevented things from getting any worse?

*If lower than previous session*: What would need to happen to move up by one point?

At what point on the scale would we know things were good enough to stop therapy?

## Worksheet 10.3

## Mapping out current skills in preparation for the therapeutic journey

Think about if you were going on a long day's walk in the hills, what might you pack? Food? Water? Compass? Map? First-aid kit? Mobile phone?

If we think about therapy like a journey, then in order to get to the point you want to get to (e.g. feeling less X or having more Y days) 'what skills do you already have that can help us on our journey?'

Use this map below to list these skills already present.

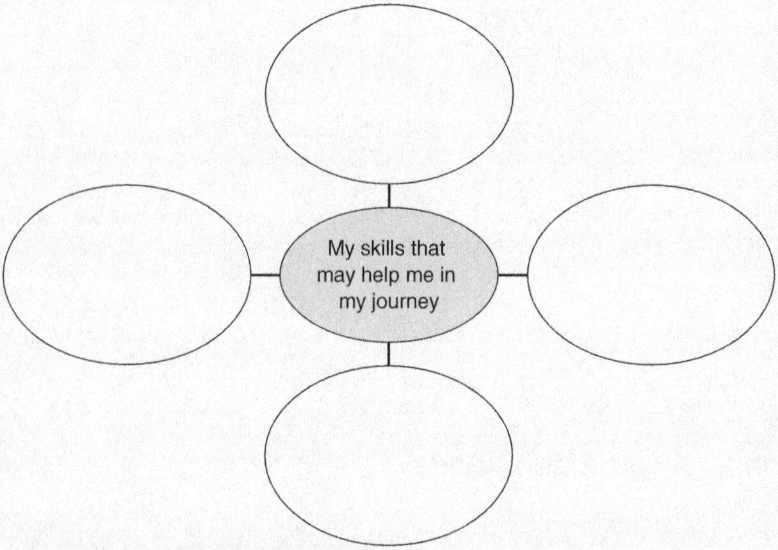


This may not be easy to think about, but here is a question that may help prompt some ideas:

> Think of a time when you have got through a tricky situation (e.g. at work, or with a friend perhaps), what skills did you use? These may have involved being: organised, disciplined, open-minded, determined, able to listen, able to draw on other people for support. Which of these may be useful to pack for our therapy journey?

# Worksheet 10.4

## Reflecting on progress

If we think about therapy as a journey, what important steps have you taken on this journey and how exactly did you manage to take them? You may have been able to make a step forward in therapy through developing a particular skill, by gaining a particular insight, or by behaving in a certain way. Use the footsteps below to map out these steps, and then think about the steps you wish to continue making once therapy has ended.

**Start of therapy:**

Step taken

How it was achieved?

Step taken

How it was achieved?

Present:

Step taken

How it was achieved?

Future:

Step taken

How will I achieve this?

# 11 DIALECTICAL BEHAVIOUR THERAPY

Phillipa Calvert

When accessing therapy it can be difficult for people to face the notion that they are 'OK' as they are, but that they may also need to change in order to achieve a 'life worth living'[1]. Dialectical behaviour therapy (DBT) utilises a combination of acceptance-based techniques and change-based techniques to achieve a balance between these two apparently opposing ideas. The model is based on an integration of a number of approaches, including cognitive behaviour therapy, ideas from Zen Buddhism and the concept of dialectics from philosophy. The therapy aims to help people regulate their emotions by developing specific skills. These skills are identified through a collaborative understanding of difficulties and possible solutions. Although the approach was originally developed for people with a diagnosis of borderline personality disorder, the ideas and techniques can be helpful when working with a variety of people.

## THE MODEL

Dialectical behaviour therapy (DBT) was developed by Marsha Linehan in the USA and grew out of her interest in frequent suicide attempts and self-harming behaviours displayed by some people accessing therapy. Linehan became increasingly involved in providing therapy to people with a diagnosis of borderline personality disorder (BPD), and it was from this work and her own personal interest in Zen Buddhism that DBT was developed. Linehan viewed the frequent overdoses as an act that was not intended to end the person's life, but a behaviour that helped the person cope in some way.

These learned behaviours may be viewed as dysfunctional, but Linehan believed that these acts were functional as a form of self-preservation. You

> For more information on using DBT in a community mental health setting with BPD, see Sampson, et al. (2006).

may recognise this type of thinking as having elements of behavioural concepts, and you would be right. DBT is considered to have behavioural ideas at its core, but also incorporates cognitive behavioural therapy (CBT) techniques, ideas from Zen Buddhism, and emphasises the need to pay close attention to the relationship between the therapist and the person.

As DBT was developed from Linehan's conceptualisation of the origins of BPD, it is helpful to spend a little time learning about these foundations because it helps to clarify the theoretical stance and the model. Linehan takes a biosocial view of BPD, acknowledging two levels that influence the development and continuation of, and displaying of, particular behaviours:

- Intrapersonal biology.
- The interpersonal social environment.

There are several factors that interact on both levels, illustrated in Figure 11.1.

The biosocial model suggests that some individuals have a biological weakness, which makes them more emotionally vulnerable. This vulnerability is influenced by the person's upbringing; for example, they may have been born into a family and/or culture that discourages or punishes the display of

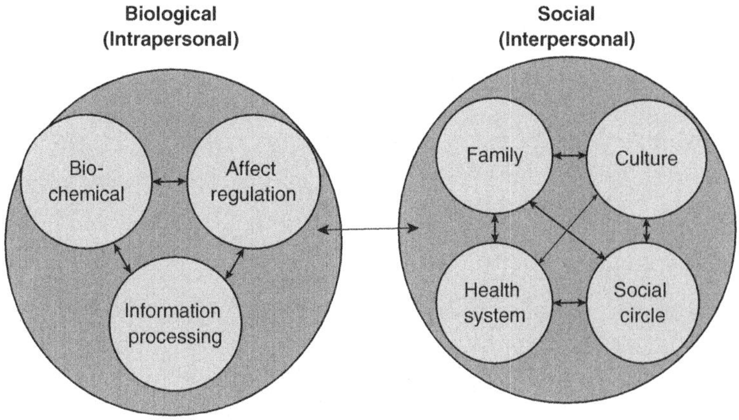


**Figure 11.1** The two levels that influence behaviour in borderline personality disorder

> If you would like to know more about the biosocial model of BPD that DBT was developed from, see Linehan (1993a) or Swales and Heard (2009).

emotion. Linehan (1993a) described this as 'an invalidating environment', whereby the individual does not have the opportunity to learn how to regulate or express their emotions, resulting in attempts to do so that can create more problems or lead to regular periods of crisis. This results in an increased sensitivity and reactivity to emotion, and greater difficulties in reducing the level of emotional arousal.

Unfortunately this pattern of invalidation can also be replicated by the health system and current social situation as the person may experience ongoing invalidation of their feelings, or feel as though they are being punished for trying to cope in the only way they know how. For example, just think about the term 'personality disorder'. The term suggests there is something fundamentally wrong with your personality, and thus with you. You are not normal, and therefore what you do is not normal. This is an example of invalidation that the individual may experience on a regular basis – but that is a whole other chapter/book. This highlights two of the main concepts in DBT:

- Difficulties in affect regulation are key to the behaviours a person engages in, and a key area for intervention.
- The person is seen to be doing the best that they can do, and not as someone who is purposefully difficult. Their behaviours make sense when looked at in context. The key is to differentiate between the person's affect on others and their intentions.

DBT attempts to validate the individual and their experiences, rather than see their behaviours as pathological and dysfunctional. The philosophical standpoint of DBT assumes that everyone is capable of understanding, having insight, and of having wisdom. Some individuals may struggle to access this capability, so the goal of therapy is to identify and develop it through a variety of means.

> The principle of dialectics was originally used by ancient philosophers to improve logic. For further reading on the use of dialectics in social psychology see Georgoudi (1983), and in the development of adult thinking, see Basseches (1984).

Another key concept in DBT is the philosophy of dialectics. The principle is that for every idea or concept (thesis), there is also an anti-thesis in direct opposition. A person can hold both;

however, as the ideas are opposing, this creates conflict and means the person can get stuck. In order for there to be change a synthesis has to be found, which allows both sides to be acknowledged and a resolution established. This allows for change to be possible and an alternative behaviour or approach to be utilised, demonstrated in Figure 11.2.

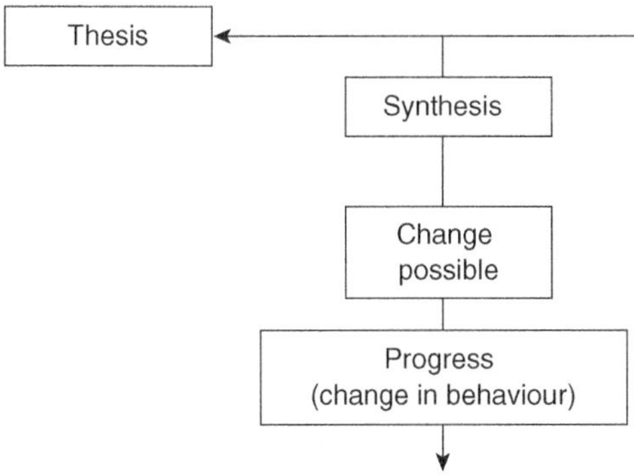


**Figure 11.2** The principle of dialectics in DBT

Dialectics can be thought of as a process that occurs for each of us to help our development, and may come into effect every time we need to make a difficult decision. In DBT this principle is used to help conceptualise the conflicts that need to be identified and resolved.

One of the main dialectic concepts in DBT is that people are acceptable as they are, but they also need to change in order to create a life worth living. The therapist balances strategies that accept the person and help make the behaviour understandable in context, but also promotes strategies to help the person alter that behaviour. The idea is that change cannot occur without acceptance, and that acceptance in itself is change. The DBT model utilises Zen principles to provide acceptance skills and CBT techniques that provide the vehicle of change. The two approaches are integrated using dialectics.

The model can be used in various settings, with a range of populations (not just BPD). Hopefully the following application section will help you think about what this looks like, or could look like, in your own therapeutic work.

## APPLICATION

DBT could be thought of as a system of therapy. The full approach involves individual therapy, group work, consultation with the person and group consultation for the therapist. Each element is designed to help implement a specific function of the approach (see Table 11.1).

| Function/aim of DBT | Element/mode of DBT delivery |
|---|---|
| Enhance capabilities | Skills group |
| Improve motivation | One-to-one therapy |
| Generalisation | Consultation to the person |
| Structure the environment | Working systemically and case management |
| Enhance therapist's skills and motivation | Consultation to the therapist |

**Table 11.1** The five functions of DBT and the corresponding mode used

This system is designed to help the person:

- Gain wisdom about their particular behaviours.
- Accept themselves but also.
- Consider change.
- Develop skills to regulate their emotions more effectively.

In turn, the system is also designed to help the therapist apply the same principles to themselves while remaining focused on the goals of therapy.

At this point you may be thinking: 'But there is no way I can do all of that in my practice!' However, remember the full DBT system was designed for individuals with quite chaotic lives, very difficult interpersonal relationships, and high levels of self-harm. There are elements of DBT that you can implement in practice with less chaotic situations (see the case study at the end of the chapter).

> Swales and Heard (2009) provide a succinct overview of the most recent research into DBT and its efficacy for women diagnosed with BPD, and other research into using DBT with substance use and binge eating.

While reading the following, try to hold in mind that the aim is to validate the person's experiences and reactions. Validation does not necessarily mean agreeing with someone's reactions or reasons, but demonstrating that these are understandable (see Worksheet 11.1 for some strategies).

## Goals of therapy

Let's start by considering what the goals are in DBT, before we look at how these are achieved. The DBT approach outlines a hierarchy of (largely pre-determined) goals, which are individualised to the person.

### Goal 1: Life-threatening behaviours

As these are considered the most dangerous behaviours that could result in significant harm to the individual, they are targeted first. These behaviours could involve self-harm, substance misuse, eating disorders or other potentially dangerous behaviours. This category also includes harm to others, such as physical aggression/violence.

> **Example:** Nem, 28, had been diagnosed with borderline personality disorder at the age of 23 following frequent admissions to hospital due to suicide attempts. Since that time she continued to experience intense and rapid changes in mood and had continued to self-harm by cutting, head-banging and swallowing bleach. Nem also continued to have frequent admissions to hospital, usually following an overdose of her prescription medication.

Once the function of these behaviours is identified, the individual is helped to acknowledge and accept these behaviours before alternative forms of coping are explored and practised.

### Goal 2: Therapy-interfering behaviours

This involves working with behaviours exhibited by both the person and the therapist. For example, the person continually misses appointments, is dissociating within the sessions or feeling angry with the therapist. Examples for the therapist include: avoiding certain topics as the person has become upset or angry; feeling resentment or frustration towards the person accessing therapy. These can prevent the therapist from accepting the person as they are, validating their experiences and exploring the barriers to change.

### Goal 3: Quality of life-interfering behaviours

This acknowledges that individuals often have an array of difficulties, possibly including other mental health diagnoses. It is recognised that even though an individual may reduce 'risky' behaviours and learn new skills in regulating their emotions, there may be other difficult experiences that continue to interfere with their life. Targeting these difficulties is thought to become possible once the individual has achieved some behavioural stability.

### Goal 4: Learning of behavioural skills

The first three aims can be achieved by increasing an individual's skills. If we consider that many of the individual's behaviours are ways of coping with difficult situations and emotions, then, in order for change to be possible, they may need new and alternative skills to manage these difficulties. New skills are gained through attending the skills group and individual one-to-one therapy.

These four goals may sound like a lot to achieve, but remember the full DBT service is not considered to be a brief intervention by modern standards. There are different modes and stages in DBT, which help work towards the goals. In the full DBT service these modes include individual therapy, skills group consultation to the person, working systemically and consultation group for the therapist.

## Individual therapy

This is typically for an hour a week. Initially this time is used to help orientate the person to the approach, including using a biosocial explanation of their current difficulties. The therapist and person negotiate specific goals for the therapy and agree on a commitment to therapy. These conversations involve elements of motivational interviewing to help the person contemplate change.

As part of this process the therapist will introduce the person to the concept of dialectics, in particular the dialectic between acceptance and change. It is also important to explore the person's own dialectic to help link their desire for change to the DBT approach. Figure 11.3 uses Nem's experience as an example.

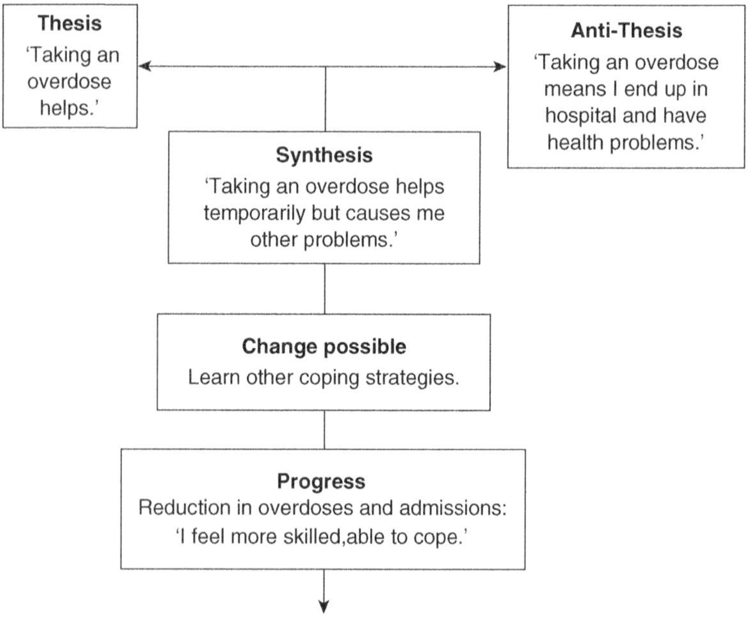


**Figure 11.3** Nem's dialectic about taking an overdose

Once a commitment to therapy has been made, the therapist will undertake a behavioural chain analysis of the 'problem' behaviours with the person and agree on solutions to help break the pattern of behaviour. The aims of the behavioural chain analysis are to identify and assess the factors that precede/elicit the behaviour and those that maintain it. This is achieved by linking the target behaviour to a trigger or activating event, emotions and the resulting consequences.

It is important to consider the consequences of the behaviour, as these are thought to reinforce the behaviour and make it more likely for the person to do it again. You may again notice the similarities between a behavioural approach and DBT. A behavioural conceptualisation would consider the link between an antecedent, behaviour and consequences in an ABC sequence as shown in Figure 11.4.

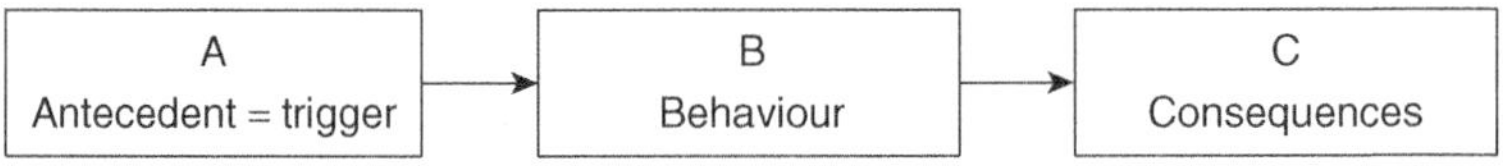


**Figure 11.4** A basic behavioural conceptualisation

DBT extends this way of conceptualising behaviour by considering occurrences that may contribute to the person being more vulnerable to a strong emotional reaction. Emotions are an important element in a DBT behavioural chain analysis and are listed as a separate link in the chain. It is also important to consider the intensity of the emotion and how the behaviour reduces the emotion, but may also result in other new emotions. This helps acknowledge that the behaviours the person engages in have a function, the main one often being to help manage their emotions.

The amount of links in a chain is individualised to the person. However, the first step in any analysis is to identify which behaviour you wish to perform the analysis on. The behaviour could be one of the life-threatening behaviours (e.g. self-harm) or it could be a therapy-interfering behaviour (e.g. not turning up to appointments). The second step is to define the problem behaviour in a non-judgemental way. The description must be specific. As an example, listing the target behaviour as 'the person acting aggressively' is too general. It would need to be broken down into specific behaviours, such as 'shouting at my partner' or 'throwing his mobile phone at the wall'. Once the behaviour has been defined, then the rest of the chain can be constructed.

Once the target behaviour has been identified it can be confusing about whether to start at the top of the chain or to work forward from the behaviour to identify the links to the consequences. There are no hard and fast rules, and the best approach is the one that makes sense to the therapist and the person accessing therapy. The next step in the analysis is to identify the links in the chain where, had the person done something differently, the problem behaviour would not have occurred. The person may not currently be able to identify what they could have done differently, and this will form part of the work in the individual session. Using Nem's case as an example Figure 11.5 illustrates the process of a behavioural chain analysis.

Once potential links to be changed have been identified, a solution analysis can be carried out. This involves the therapist and person generating potential solutions to help break the chain that leads to the behaviour. Several alternative solutions to one link can be generated and may involve developing new or reinforcing current skills. It is important that any potential obstacles are identified. This can provide an opportunity to problem-solve and practice the skills in session through role-play and rehearsal.

**Example:** Zoe came to therapy for help in managing her depression and anger outbursts at home. Through conducting a behavioural chain analysis relating to a recent anger outburst at home, Zoe identified that her fear of her partner 'finding someone else' had led to a heated argument after he returned home from a night out. This led Zoe and her therapist to discuss skills in distress tolerance and mindfulness as possible solutions to these links in the chain.

The process of the behavioural chain analysis and solution analysis helps the person to develop an understanding of their difficulties. It also considers how emotions are related to events, and the function of subsequent behaviours. Finally, it helps the therapist discuss the role of a skills group in helping the person develop new skills (see Worksheet 11.4).

Individual therapy continues in conjunction with the skills group, and the therapist aims to help the person apply the new skills they are learning and individualise them to the person. The therapist encourages and models to the person a way of looking at their life in a non-judgemental and more compassionate way. In this way the person can start to develop wisdom about their lives and recognise their role in the problems they are experiencing.

## Skills group

Some quick points regarding the skills group:

- Usually consisting of 6–8 people (but can be just two people plus the facilitators), of mixed gender and is typically two and a half hours per week.

| Link in chain | What is this? | Nem's example |
| --- | --- | --- |
| Vulnerabilities | Things that might make the person more susceptible to reacting emotionally. | *Lack of sleep and not eating during days as hoping to go for meal with boyfriend.* |
| Trigger/activating event | The specific event that seemed to set off the chain. The point where things seemed to start from. | *Nem's boyfriend arriving home late having already eaten and saying he forgot they were meant to be going out to eat.* |
| Emotion (and intensity) | The person's emotional reaction to the event. There might be more than one emotion. | *Nem felt very upset – rated as 4/5 on her emotional reaction scale.* |
| Anything else? | Any other important details that would link the event to the behaviour.This might be thoughts or physical feelings. | *Nem experienced thoughts about her boyfriend not loving her and wanting to leave her.* |
| Target behaviour | A description of the specific behaviour that the person wants to change. | *When her boyfriend went to bed Nem went into the bathroom and used one of his razors to cut the tops of her arms.* |
| Emotion (and intensity) | The person's emotions immediately after the event. Looking for a change in emotion. | *Nem had felt a sense of relief and rated the upset as 2/5.* |
| Anything else? | Any other important details that would link the behaviour to the consequences. | *Afterwards Nem had felt a deep sense of shame about the cutting and reported 'telling herself off'.* |
| Consequences | The outcome of the behaviour. There can be more than one consequence. | *Her boyfriend then came into the bathroom and shouted at her, telling her that she was being manipulative, leaving her feeling upset.* |

**Figure 11.5** Flow chart of Nem's behavioural chain analysis

- Based on a psychoeducation approach rather than group therapy.
- Consideration given to each person before organising for them to attend a mixed-gender group, as some people may have experienced physical or sexual abuse.
- Aim is to help the person learn the necessary skills to develop alternative and more helpful ways of regulating their emotions and managing relationships.
- Covers four modules: core mindfulness, distress tolerance, emotion regulation; and interpersonal effectiveness.
- The person is often expected to complete each module twice over a year to optimise their learning opportunities, practice their new skills and receive support while implementing them in their daily lives.
- There are typically two facilitators who run the group, helping the attendees to learn new skills. As a facilitator it is important to be aware of group processes, but these are not explored within the group.

> Linehan's website has some diary card examples under 'Tools for Clinicians' at www.behaviouraltech.org.

Each session follows roughly the same format each week. Typically the homework from the previous week is reviewed, including any queries or difficulties each individual experienced. A new skill is then discussed, which builds on the skills previously learnt. Homework is set based on this new skill, and group members are encouraged to identify potential opportunities for using the skill and any possible obstacles. Some groups complete a mindfulness exercise at the beginning of each session, regardless of the current module, prior to reviewing the homework. Others also review the diary card to help the person recognise the skills they have used during the week and also provide positive feedback to the individual for attempting to use the skills they have been learning. This tends to be when a full DBT service is not set up and the person may therefore only have access to the skills group and not the individual therapy.

The modules and indeed each session are described in detail in Linehan's (1993b) skills manual. However, to give you a flavour, the purpose and content of each module is briefly outlined below.

## Core mindfulness

DBT introduces mindfulness as a skill, which may seem to go against the idea that mindfulness is not about doing, it is about being. DBT argues that individuals need to learn the skill and thus need to 'do' before they can 'be'. Linehan introduced the concept of 'wisemind' as part of the DBT application of mindfulness. Wisemind is described as a 'balance between feelings and

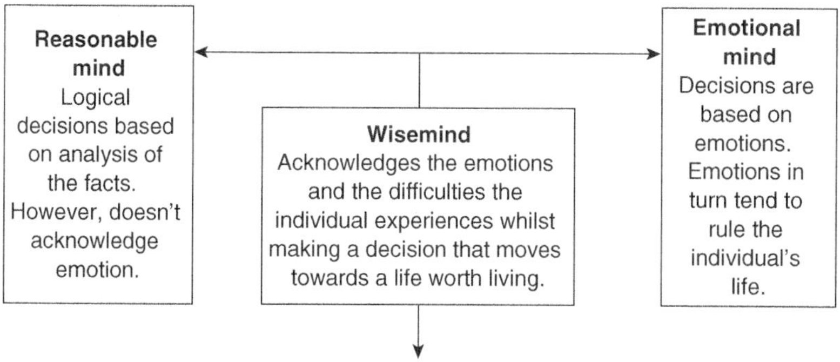


**Figure 11.6** The concept of reasonable mind, emotional mind and wisemind in DBT

rational thoughts' (McKay, et al. 2007: 87). Wisemind has been likened to intuition, and can be thought of as a synthesis between emotional mind and reasonable mind (see Figure 11.6).

> **Example:** Zoe identified that she often acted in emotional mind and felt that her emotions took over. She struggled to 'think things through'. Practising mindfulness on a daily basis helped Zoe to not get caught up in the emotion, or her thoughts, and tune into her intuition rather than her fear that her partner would leave.

### Distress tolerance

This module aims to help individuals recognise emotions, which they often experience as overwhelming. Individuals have often struggled to manage these emotions in effective ways (e.g. using substances, taking out distress on others, avoidance). Distress tolerance skills therefore focus on skills that are deemed to be more helpful and adaptive, such as distraction, self-soothing and radical acceptance.

### Emotional regulation

Individuals who struggle with overwhelming emotions can also struggle to recognise their emotions, often saying things like 'I feel awful' or 'It's just a mess'. In DBT a distinction is made between primary emotions and secondary emotions. Primary emotions are the initial emotional reactions to an event, for example anxiety at the prospect of having to drive on the motorway after an accident. Secondary emotions are a reaction to the primary emotion. So in the same example, someone may start to feel depressed about how anxious they feel. This can quickly snowball and emotions become entangled creating a mess of feelings.

Emotion regulation skills are therefore designed to help people to:

- Understand more about emotions.
- Be able to recognise and name emotions.
- Expose the individual to both difficult and pleasant emotions.
- Problem-solve.
- Learn to recognise emotional urges and develop alternative responses.

### Interpersonal effectiveness

The focus here is to develop an individual's skills in expressing their needs and beliefs in a way that is respectful to both the individual and the people they are interacting with. It is also about problem-solving in social situations, and helping individuals to set boundaries for friendships and relationships.

> **Example:** Zoe was reluctant at first to try out any of the assertiveness skills or ideas for discussing how she felt with her partner. She discussed this with her therapist and they agreed to practise the skills in session and set less challenging examples as homework to build up her confidence. Zoe and the therapist then practised Zoe talking about some of her feelings with her partner through role-play.

So, now that we have looked at the individual therapy and skills group aspects of DBT, let's consider consultation to the person, systemic working and the consultation group for the therapist.

## Consultation to the person

This can be one of the most challenging elements of DBT as it involves the person contacting the therapist in between sessions and out of hours, something which might seem very daunting. The aim of consultation is to help the person think about the new skill they are learning and trying to apply it in their everyday lives. This recognises that generalisation from the therapy to everyday life does not always happen automatically. The person is encouraged to seek consultation at times when they recognise a familiar pattern is occurring, but importantly *before* a crisis. This allows the therapist and person to generate a possible solution, select an appropriate skill and think about how they will practice this.

The format of consultation to the person can vary depending on the setting. When the person is on a mental health ward, a member of staff on each shift would be identified as the coach who can provide on-the-spot consultation. When the person is accessing the DBT service as an outpatient, they are given a phone number. This is where a team approach is useful, so the responsibility of providing the consultation is shared.

## Working systemically

This is structuring the environment for the person, including the therapy approach, clinical services providing input to the person, and the systems around the person in their everyday life (Swales and Heard, 2009). If we think about the biosocial model of BPD, it suggests that an invalidating environment cannot only contribute to but also maintain the difficulties the individual experiences. This would suggest that there needs to be interventions at this level to help the system around the individual adjust to, facilitate and reinforce the new skills they are trying to use.

Working towards structuring the environment the person lives in could be done through meetings held as part of the care programme approach (CPA), with family, carers and support staff. The aim is to help other people be aware of their own behaviour, and how this might unwittingly reinforce unhelpful behaviours in the person accessing therapy.

## Consultation group for the therapist

The consultation group could be likened to group supervision, but is quite structured and aims to help maintain the therapist's motivation and application of DBT. It is recommended that the consultation group is held weekly for approximately two hours. It has training elements, to help develop the therapist's skills. It also aims to help the therapist identify their own therapy-interfering behaviours. Some of the techniques used with the person accessing therapy are also utilised in the consultation group.

## Organisation of DBT

As you have probably gathered, offering a full DBT service requires a great deal of coordination and support from the wider service that the programme sits in. The final practical aspect of applying DBT is to consider how this is organised and in what order everything happens. As mentioned above, DBT is organised into stages. Linehan originally proposed four stages. This was then expanded by Swales et al. (2000) to include a fifth stage (see Table 11.2).

Hopefully this chapter has helped demystify DBT and started you thinking about elements of the approach that may be useful in your own practice. Remember that while we have presented the whole DBT system intervention, it can be applied in isolation through one-to-one therapy, as illustrated in the case study.

| Stage and aim of stage | Tasks | Mode(s) |
|---|---|---|
| **Pre-treatment**<br>Establishing a collaborative understanding of the person's difficulties, identifying solutions and linking these to DBT approach. | • Introduce treatment model.<br>• Build therapeutic relationship.<br>• Develop understanding of difficulties.<br>• Explore expectations of therapy.<br>• Mutual commitment to therapy by person and therapist.<br>• Introduce dialectical stance.<br>• Link risk behaviours and targets to work on, to targets of therapy. | • One-to-one therapy.<br>• Consultation to therapist. |
| **Stage 1**<br>Achieve behavioural stability. | • Reduce immediate risk of life-threatening behaviours to self and/or others.<br>• Reduce therapy-interfering behaviours.<br>• Reduce behaviours that interfere with quality of life.<br>• Increase behavioural skills. | • Skills group.<br>• One-to-one therapy.<br>• Telephone coaching.<br>• Consultation to therapist. |
| **Stage 2**<br>Emotional processing of the past. | • Reduce any PTSD-like symptoms.<br>• Employ skills learnt in stage one. | • One-to-one therapy. |
| **Stage 3**<br>Assist people to obtain and maintain regular levels of emotion. | • Target other difficulties, such as marital, education or employment.<br>• Increase self-respect and self-validation.<br>• Continue working towards a life worth living. | These two stages are typically not offered as part of the DBT service, or addressed through the NHS.<br>Having said this, they could be achieved through:<br>• One-to-one therapy.<br>• Employment services.<br>• Voluntary organisation therapy services. |
| **Stage 4**<br>Enhance capacity for joy. | • Resolving existential issues of life. | |

**Table 11.2** The stages, tasks and modes used at each stage of DBT

## CASE STUDY

Hannah, 35, was referred by her GP due to difficulties with sleeping, fluctuating mood, anger, increasing use of alcohol, and binge eating. She had recently been assessed by a psychiatrist due to expressing thoughts of suicide. The psychiatrist had identified that Hannah had experienced at least three different times in her life when she would have met the diagnostic criteria for major depression. The current period of low mood had occurred after her husband had been involved in an accident at work, which had left him paralysed from the waist down. They have no children and no other family. At the time of the accident Hannah had just undergone a shoulder replacement that had limited her physical activities and ability to provide the physical aspects of her husband's care. The psychiatrist had diagnosed her with recurrent depressive disorder and had recommended that she was referred for psychological therapy.

Hannah described herself as a strong, independent woman who prided herself on being there for people. She was unsure about psychological therapy due to concerns about opening up Pandora's box and becoming unravelled, leaving her unable to look after her husband. However, she also described being desperate for help, recognising that she was struggling to hold things together. She confirmed experiencing some thoughts of ending her life, but had no plan or timescale. Hannah described tending to 'run on adrenaline'; she would spend days and sometimes weeks completing tasks, filling her day with activities, and mainly focusing on the needs of others and caring for her now disabled husband. She tended to 'put on a mask' to the world to ensure that others perceived her as OK and coping, but underneath she was struggling.

She found maintaining this level of activity increasingly difficult and would start to feel overwhelmed by the demands of other people. She would become more irritable, angry and aggressive, but feel guilty afterwards. Her sleep and mood would start to decrease and she would start to feel depressed and could experience suicidal thoughts. This would last for a few days, where she would hide away from the world, struggling to manage how she was feeling and trying to cope by binge eating and using alcohol. After a few days she would start to feel a bit better and feel the need to complete the tasks she had not done while feeling down. She would then return to the previous state of running on adrenaline, and the pattern would repeat.

*(Continued)*

*(Continued)*

Hannah was introduced to the idea of dialectics to explore her apparent conflicting statements regarding therapy. On the one hand, Hannah was expressing a belief that she had to keep her thoughts and feelings bottled up in order to get by, yet, on the other hand, felt that she needed help. This helped facilitate a conversation about her fears about entering therapy, and a possible way forward of developing new skills to understand and manage her emotions.

The initial sessions were dedicated to developing behavioural chain analyses, helping link Hannah's behaviours to specific emotions and triggers. This identified that Hannah would take on a lot of responsibility, struggling to say 'no' as she did not want to let anyone down. She would then become anxious about trying to manage all of the tasks she had to complete. This led to an increase in physical arousal, and irritability. Hannah would then 'snap' and become aggressive. Afterwards she tended to ruminate and found it difficult to switch off. This led to difficulties with sleeping and low mood. Hannah found it difficult to tolerate these emotions and used food and alcohol to cope and 'self-medicate'.

This helped Hannah and the therapist to identify some potential solutions:

1. Reducing the amount of tasks and responsibility, for example by agreeing to carers helping with her husband's physical needs.
2. Assertiveness skills to help her say 'no' and to increase her interpersonal skills.
3. Mindfulness skills to help her not to get caught up in the rumination.
4. Distress tolerance skills to help her manage her emotions.
5. Cognitive strategies to help challenge her self-critical thoughts and meta-cognitions about the emotions she was experiencing and her behaviour.

The remainder of the sessions were spent focusing on each of these solutions by exploring the skills Hannah already had and those she felt she needed to develop. Hannah was given homework based on the skill she was learning, and any difficulties with motivation or application of the skill was discussed during the next session. Hannah found the process difficult at times as she found talking about her experiences distressing, and she would talk about ending the therapy. This allowed the therapist to explore the dialectic outlined in Figure 11.7, validate her experiences and rediscover the commitment to change.

By the end of therapy Hannah had attended 14 sessions. She continued to report fluctuations in her mood, but was able to recognise that this was a reaction to the stressful events in her life and the role of rumination and invalidating self-critical thoughts. Hannah reported a reduction in aggressive outbursts, improvement in sleep and an increased sense of being able to cope. Her husband had commented that she seemed more relaxed and they had started to talk about the recent events and how it had affected their relationship. This is something they had avoided doing since the accident.

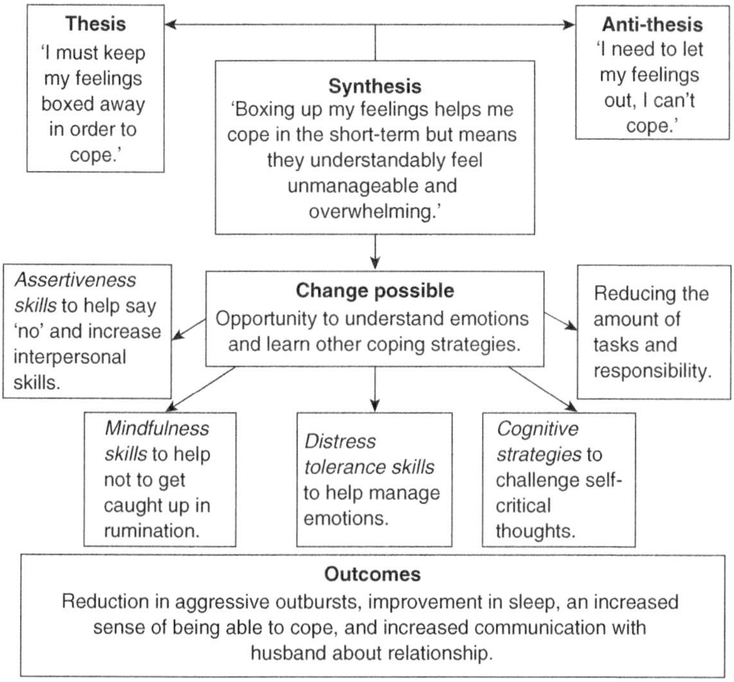


**Figure 11.7** Hannah's dialectic regrarding therapy

## GLOSSARY

A life worth living — This is a key phrase in DBT. The idea is to help individuals think about what they would like their lives to look like, and thus what would need to be different. It is not about identifying a perfect life, but one that is good enough.

Acceptance — This can be thought of as a passive act whereby the person just resigns to something. However, acceptance

| | |
|---|---|
| | in a therapeutic context is about acknowledgement without approval or judgement. I find it helpful to think about the following philosophy: 'The world cannot be any different because it was created by what has preceded it' (Aitken, 1982). |
| Affect | Another word for emotion. |
| Anti-thesis | A concept or idea that is the direct opposite of another concept or idea (thesis). |
| Automatic | Something that happens without conscious control. Thoughts can be thought of becoming automatic when they pop into your head while you are not choosing for this to happen. |
| Behavioural chain analysis | The process of linking a person's behaviour to a specific event/trigger, emotions and consequences. |
| Behavioural concepts | Relates to behaviour theory and therapy. The main focus is someone's behaviour, i.e., what they do. Behaviours are thought to occur in relation to events both as a reaction and as a way of dealing with that event. |
| Biosocial model | A theory that offers an understanding based on a combination of biology and social interactions. |
| Dialectics | The concept that everything is made of two opposing ideas or forces. The process in dialectics is to bring together these two opposing forces to bring about change. |
| Dissociate | When the person is 'here but not here'. They can appear to be cut off. You may have experienced this whilst talking to someone, when you realise you haven't been listening or were daydreaming. Dissociation can be thought to occur along a continuum, from mild to extreme as is seen in dissociative identity disorder. |
| Emotionally vulnerable | This idea stems from the biosocial model, where an individual is thought to be vulnerable to emotions and may therefore experience very intense emotions and struggle to reduce the intensity of the emotion as quickly as other people. |
| Hierarchy | A list of behaviours or goals that are organised in terms of importance, or difficulty, and used to work on in therapy. |
| Interpersonal effectiveness | A set of skills taught to help the person express their needs more effectively to other people, and to manage social situations and relationships in a way where they |

| | |
|---|---|
| | feel in control but do not become controlling. It is similar to assertiveness and social skills. |
| Intrapersonal | Something that happens within the person; for example, thoughts, physical feelings and emotions. |
| Radical acceptance | Accepting the moment for what it is, no judgement, no criticism, but an observation of what is happening now. |
| Synthesis | The bringing together of a thesis and anti-thesis. |
| Systemic | Refers to taking into account interactions between people and between different organisations when thinking about a person's problems. It also refers to working in a way that does not just focus on the individual but also on the other people and organisations that are involved in the person's life. |
| Thesis | An idea or concept. |
| Wisemind | Likened to intuition; emotions, and the difficulties the individual experiences, are acknowledged whilst making a decision that moves towards a life worth living. |

## REFERENCES

Aitken, R. (1982) *Taking the Path of Zen*. San Francisco, CA: North Point.

Basseches, M. (1984) *Dialectical Thinking and Adult Development*. Norwood, NJ: Ablex.

Georgoudi, M. (1983) 'Modern dialectics in social psychology: A reappraisal', *European Journal of Social Psychology, 13*(1), 77–93.

Linehan, M. M. (1993a) *Cognitive-behavioural Treatment of Borderline Personality Disorder*. New York: Guilford. See also www.behaviouraltech.org

Linehan, M. M. (1993b) *Skills Training Manual for Treating Borderline Personality Disorder*. New York: Guilford.

McKay, M., Wood, J. C. and Brantley, J. (2007) *The Dialectical Behaviour Therapy Skills Workbook*. Oakland, CA: New Harbinger.

Sampson, M. J., McCubbin, R. A. and Tyrer, P. (2006) *Personality Disorder and Community Mental Health Teams: A Practitioner's Guide*. Chichester: Wiley.

Swales, M. A. and Heard, H. L. (2009) *Dialectical Behaviour Therapy: The CBT Distinctive Features Series*. New York: Routledge.

Swales, M. A., Heard, H. L. and Williams, J. G. (2000) 'Linehan's dialectical behaviour therapy (DBT) for borderline personality disorder: Overview and adaptation', *Journal of Mental Health, 9*, 7–23.

## NOTE

1. This might seem like a strange term, but it is a key phrase in the DBT approach. It refers to the way a person would like their life to be (not necessarily a perfect life, but a better one).

# Worksheet 11.1

## Validation strategies

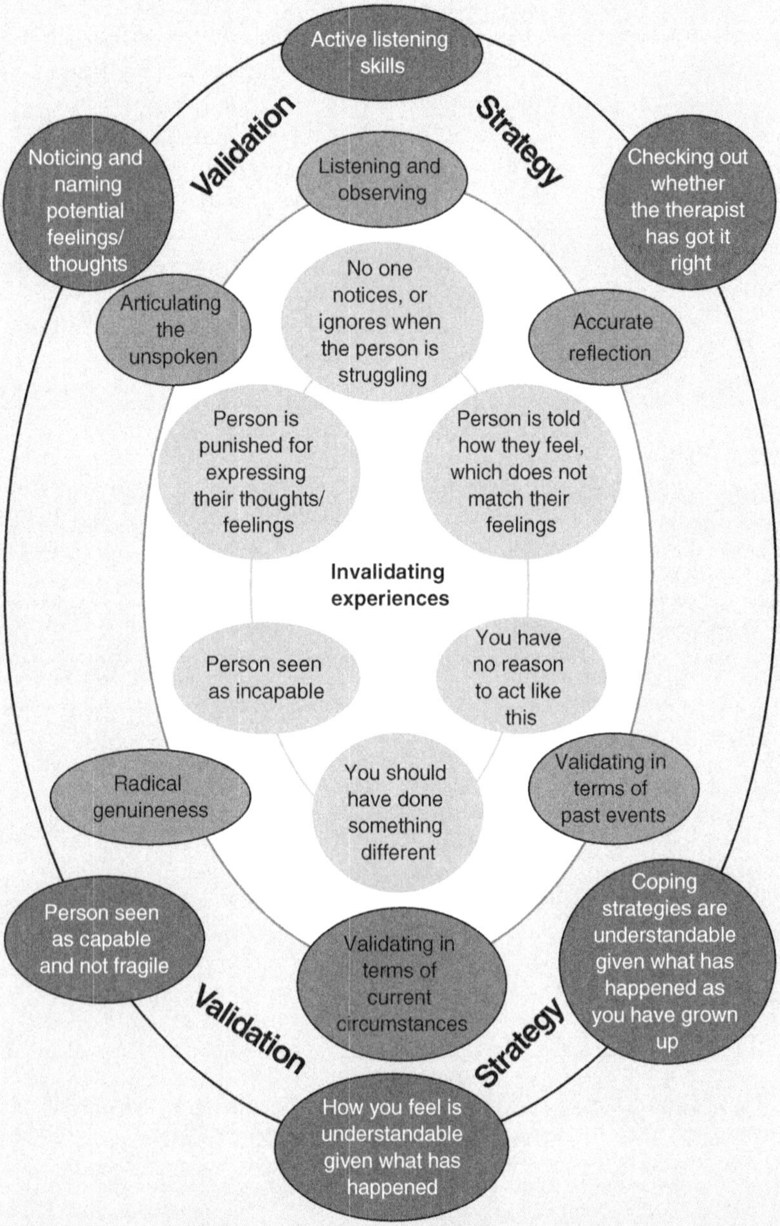

# Worksheet 11.2

## Balancing acceptance and change

This worksheet will hopefully help you think about the potentially difficult balance between acceptance and change.

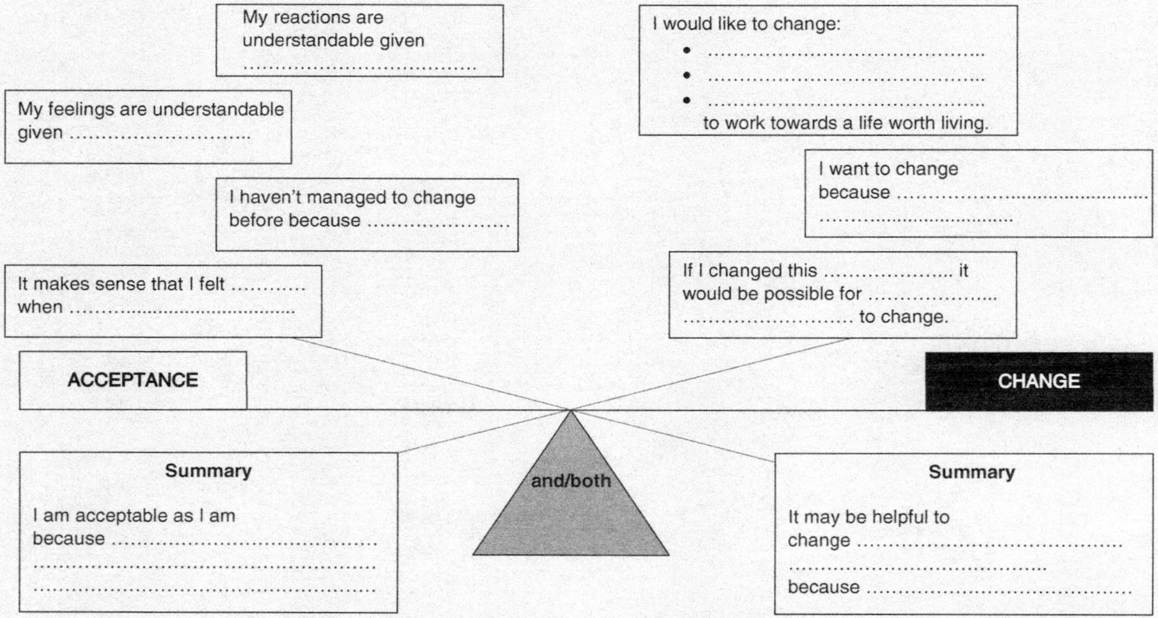

# Worksheet 11.3

## Dialectics

This worksheet will hopefully help you think about some common dialectics that occur for people. There is also some space at the end of the sheet to enter your own. The first two contain a synthesis, but the rest have been left blank for you to enter your own thoughts on a possible synthesis.

| | | |
|---|---|---|
| **Acceptance** 'I am acceptable as I am.' | **Synthesis** 'I am OK and a worthwhile person who could learn new skills to help change aspects of my life I struggle with.' | **Change** 'I have to change.' |
| **Logic** 'I have to be rational in my decisions.' | **Synthesis** 'I can recognise my emotions and think about why something may be difficult for me but choose what to do.' | **Emotion** 'My emotions rule my life and my decisions.' |
| **Independence** 'I have to be self-sufficient and not rely on anyone.' | **Synthesis** | **Dependence** 'I cannot cope on my own and need others to do everything.' |
| **Control** 'I have to plan everything and be prepared.' | **Synthesis** | **Improvise** 'I wing it which gives me freedom but means chaos.' |
| | | |

# Worksheet 11.4

## Example behavioural chain analysis and possible solutions

| Questions to ask | Chain | Possible solutions |
|---|---|---|
| Has anything been different recently? Sleep, medication, physical health? | Vulnerabilities | |
| What was happening immediately before I did the target behaviour? Who was there, what happened, where did it happen, what time? | Trigger/activating event | |
| How did you feel? Is this the emotion that happened right after the event? How intense was it? Use a 0 (none) – 5 (very intense) rating scale. | Emotion (and intensity) | |
| Did you have any thoughts about the feelings you were having? Or about the activating event? Any other details that might be important? | Anything else? | |
| What did you do? To who? Where were you? When did it happen? What time did it happen? | Target Behaviour | |
| How did you feel immediately afterwards? How intense was it? Use a 0 (none) – 5 (very intense) rating scale. | Emotion (and intensity) | |
| Did you have any thoughts about the feelings you were having? Or about the activating event? Any other details that might be important? | Anything else? | |
| What happened afterwards? How did other people react immediately and later? What effect did the behaviour have on you? | Consequences | |

# 12 OUTCOMES IN THERAPY

Stephen Weatherhead and
Graeme Flaherty-Jones

Talking therapies, regardless of their philosophical underpinning, and practical application should be considering whether or not they are useful to those who access therapy. In this final chapter, we discuss how to define what an outcome is, and various ways in which to measure outcomes. We highlight some of the factors that influence how to select, gather and disseminate different forms of evidence in therapy.

## WHAT ARE OUTCOMES?

Outcome measurement is one of those topics that seems to cycle into and out of the awareness of therapists, and others who have a part to play in therapy. At times of financial constraints it is particularly important, probably because if pennies are being counted then expenditure needs to have tangible justification. At other times there is less focus on the outcome of therapy, and more on the philosophy and practice of the approach. Within this chapter, we attempt to balance therapeutic philosophy (epistemology) with the viewpoint that we all have a moral responsibility to somehow capture whether what we are doing is useful.

We'll tread through the philosophical minefield of how best to capture usefulness a little later, but for now let's assume the following: the outcome of any therapeutic intervention is best evidenced in relation to the goals that therapy sets itself. Feltham (2006) defined 12 possible goals of therapy (see Table 12.1).

Unfortunately, evidencing therapeutic outcome is not straightforward, even if we can agree on the goal of any given therapy. If only it were as simple as selecting one of the 12 goals, and picking up the corresponding outcome tool in the fashion of 'for goal A use tool B'. There is an ever-growing number of ways to evidence outcome, all of which are open to epistemological and logistical criticisms, and none

> What do you personally think is the best way to show whether therapy has been useful?

| | |
|---|---|
| 1. | **Support**<br>As it says on the tin: providing unconditional regard for the person(s) accessing therapy. |
| 2. | **Psycho-educational guidance**<br>Helping a person develop skills to better understand their situation, and manage its impact. |
| 3. | **Adjustment and resource provision**<br>Providing tangible information/tools to assist a person in accepting their circumstances. |
| 4. | **Crisis intervention and management**<br>Guiding those accessing services through particularly challenging situations, and back to where they were before the crisis occurred. |
| 5. | **Problem-solving and decision making**<br>Developing practical solutions to contextual problems. |
| 6. | **Symptom amelioration**<br>Reducing specific, measurable phenomena. |
| 7. | **Insight and Understanding**<br>Uncovering the reasons behind a problem developing and conceptualising the factors that maintain it. |
| 8. | **Cure**<br>Completely eliminating the problem. |
| 9. | **Self-actualisation**<br>Helping the person to gain a greater understanding of their self, and working towards the preferred version of that self. |
| 10. | **Personality change**<br>Changing a person's life to the extent that they feel that they have shifted at the very core of who they are. |
| 11. | **Discovery of meaning and transcendental experience**<br>Evoking change on a spiritual/philosophical level. |
| 12. | **Systemic, organisational or social change**<br>Changing the interactions/perspectives of a group of people. |

**Table 12.1** Twelve goals of therapy (adapted from Feltham, 2006: 11–16)

of which are universally accepted by all proponents of the relevant model (never mind the therapeutic world as a whole).

Even defining what an outcome is can be a difficult thing. The term 'outcomes' has different meanings to different people. For some it is all about complying with legislative guidelines, and 'gold standard' research founded in randomised controlled trials. For others it is about a change in individual stories and a shift in emphasis. For most people, be they commissioners, therapists or a person in the street thinking of accessing therapy, it is simply about reducing the impact of a problem. The real challenge comes when trying to capture/evidence whether the therapeutic process has been useful in meeting this aim.

## HOW TO MEASURE OUTCOMES

A seminal text by Lambert (1992) found that the therapeutic model itself may only account for 15 per cent of the change that occurs. The rest is accounted for by the therapeutic relationship, the expectations of the person accessing therapy, and 'client factors', which can be defined as a person's individual resources (e.g. ego strength and social support) (see Figure 12.1).

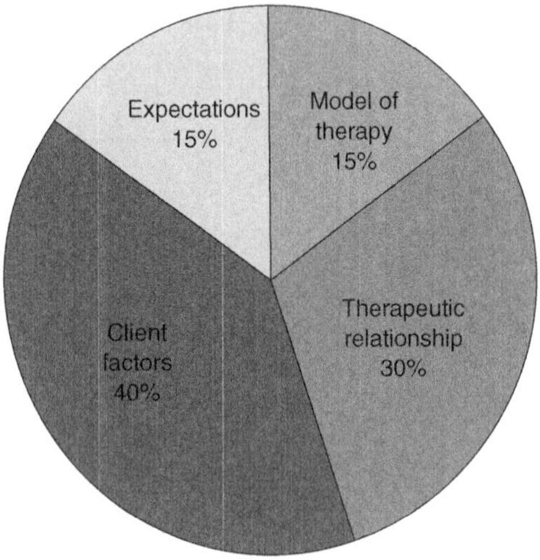


**Figure 12.1** The therapeutic model after (Lambert, 1992)

One approach to evidencing outcomes could be to take each component of this model separately. Beginning with 'client factors', we have first to accept that it's quite difficult to assess all the different facets that make up what Lambert (1992) describes as client factors. However, some therapeutic models do focus directly on them within the techniques used. For example, systemic therapies and dialectical behaviour therapy often include family members, and psychodynamic therapy for example, pays attention to ego strength. Other therapy approaches focus on them in a more indirect manner, for example solution-focused brief therapy and cognitive behavioural therapy encourage the person to consider what they bring to therapy and find solutions to the problem, and mindfulness supports a person in developing techniques to become more deliberate in their responses to situations.

Therefore, whilst they are termed 'client factors', therapeutic interventions can still have a part to play in helping reduce their role in psychological difficulties. However, given that it is difficult to gain a comprehensive understanding of all the facets of a person's individual resources prior to therapy, it is perhaps even more difficult to fully evidence their change afterwards.

A significant challenge is also posed when it comes to evaluating the role of expectations and 'the placebo effect'. According to this model, it accounts for as much of the outcome as the therapeutic approach itself. Most therapies would advocate discussing what people are expecting or hoping for when they access therapy, but what it is virtually impossible to capture is the level of those expectations, and how that influences outcome.

This all seems quite pessimistic so far, but it's not all doom and gloom. Let's have a quick look at the section described as the 'therapeutic relationship'. You will have noticed that the Lambert model suggests that the therapeutic relationship can account for up to 30 per cent of the outcome of therapy. In the introductory chapter, you will have read about what the therapeutic relationship is, how to maintain it, and what its role is in therapy. Capturing this to form an outcome measure is quite difficult. However, it's not impossible – most therapies have attempted to do so. Unfortunately it's not easy to tease them out as they are referred to in a range of ways, such as 'session rating scales', 'process measures' and 'working alliance measures'.

As you might expect, each therapeutic model has its own perspective on evidencing the utility of therapy, and very few of them would say that they are only considering the 15 per cent allocated to the 'model of therapy' in the pie chart shown in Figure 12.1. Furthermore, they all have their own language, form and ways of disseminating outcome evidence. Table 12.2 shows a selection of the many techniques that we as therapists could consider in our own practice.

These are just a small selection of the ways in which therapy can be evaluated and outcomes gathered. You will notice that there is no column indicating the type of therapy for which each form of evidence is most appropriate. This is because it is an evolving landscape, which we as therapists have a role in shaping. The selection of outcome evidence is influenced by many factors, as shown in the next section, as is the way in which that evidence is shared with the people involved (e.g. through publications, research, presentations, letters).

## THE PHILOSOPHY OF EVIDENCING OUTCOMES

We've looked at what outcomes are and how they can be evidenced; next we consider some of the factors that influence these issues. Let's

| Form of evidence | Description | Pros and cons |
| --- | --- | --- |
| **Standardised questionnaires** | Questionnaires that have been researched to ensure that they are accurate in assessing any given phenomena.<br>They are often symptom-focused, and look at a specific issue such as depression, anxiety, hopelessness. | **Pros:**<br>They are respected amongst the wider community.<br>They provide a straightforward before and after comparison.<br>They are often quite easy to administer, and sometimes come in short forms that don't take much time to complete.<br>**Cons:**<br>They are unable to fully capture a person's experience.<br>They are often revised, and go out of date.<br>They can be relatively expensive.<br>They often require a certain level of ability to complete.<br>The language used can be inconsistent with many therapeutic models. |
| **Process measures*** | Assessments focused on identifying the specific factors that have influenced change during therapy.<br>Also referred to as 'session ratings scales' or 'working alliance scales'. | **Pros:**<br>They don't just focus on whether therapy was useful, but also consider which aspects were useful.<br>They provide an opportunity to engage with the debate around outcome evidence, without necessarily conforming to the dominant view.<br>**Cons:**<br>They are often tailored to a particular model.<br>They do not fully show whether therapy has been effective with its intended purpose of reducing the problem. |
| **Quality of life measures*** | Questionnaires that consider different aspects that can affect a person's overall wellbeing.<br>Common factors assessed often include health, community engagement, employment, social life, leisure activities, psychological wellbeing. | **Pros:**<br>They capture some of the holistic aspects of a person's experience.<br>**Cons:**<br>They are often culture-specific, and make a lot of assumptions about what constitutes quality of life. |
| **Service satisfaction assessments** | Questionnaires that assess how pleased a person is with the service they have received. | **Pros:**<br>They provide a good base for assessing what needs to change about service provision.<br>They capture a more general attitude-based view on the therapy participated in, and its general utility. |

*(Continued)*

*(Continued)*

| Form of evidence | Description | Pros and cons |
| --- | --- | --- |
| | | **Cons:**<br>They are difficult to standardise, and as such have limited generalisability.<br>Service satisfaction does not necessarily mean that the therapy achieved its goals. |
| **Non-standardised questionnaires** | An individualised set of questions focused on the topics that are particularly important to the person accessing therapy.<br>They can be developed collaboratively between the therapist and the person accessing therapy. | **Pros:**<br>They can be tailored to the needs and ability of those involved in therapy.<br>They provide a personal view on things in a way that standardised questionnaires can't.<br>**Cons:**<br>They are only applicable to the individual themselves, and so cannot be widely administered.<br>They are not detailed enough to fully capture the intricacies of therapy.<br>Goals often change during therapy, so it can be difficult to gauge pre and post changes. |
| **Skills-based assessments*** | These focus on a person's ability to complete a given task.<br>Examples include their ability to engage in employment, or take care of themselves. | **Pros:**<br>The task-related focus can be quite empowering.<br>They provide a clear structure.<br>They take into account a person's individual circumstances.<br>**Cons:**<br>They don't really apply to a lot of therapies, and services.<br>They don't capture the qualitative aspects of therapy.<br>They don't consider a person's psychological wellbeing. |
| **Interviews** | Discussions with the person accessing therapy.<br>They can be conducted by the therapist or an independent person.<br>They can take place at different points in the therapy process.<br>They can follow set questions or be less structured. | **Pros:**<br>They allow for a full discussion of as many aspects of therapy as needed.<br>They give lots of room for the person who has accessed therapy to express their own views, in their own way.<br>**Cons:**<br>They can be quite time-consuming.<br>They can feel like a part of therapy, rather than an evaluation of it.<br>They require a lot of analysis. |

**Table 12.2** Some techniques for use in practice

* These could be either standardised or non-standardised, and as such share the same critiques.

begin by taking a look at the example below of Patrick, and consider some of the possible ways of evidencing whether therapeutic intervention has been useful.

> **Example:** Patrick is a 42-year-old man who was referred for therapy by his general practitioner. Patrick is reported to have 'longstanding depression' since his wife died three years ago. He has been off work for almost six months, no longer socialises with his friends, has a lot of trouble sleeping, and has begun having some fleeting suicidal thoughts.

Any of the 12 goals for therapy listed earlier could be perfectly appropriate to Patrick's situation. Equally, any of the ten models of therapy we have covered in this book could be justifiable interventions. In fact, as the pie chart in Figure 12.1 shows, the choice of therapy may actually play a limited role in outcome (Lambert, 1992).

Let's assume, as is often the case, that Patrick himself states quite simply 'I just don't want to feel this way anymore'. How would we capture whether therapy has been useful in meeting these aims? Here are just four of the many options available to capture this as an intended outcome:

1. **Ask Patrick to complete a standardised questionnaire or series of questionnaires:** The questionnaire(s) would usually be administered before therapy began, then again afterwards, then possibly again sometime later (pre, post, follow-up). The questionnaires could be self report and/or completed by an independent rater (e.g. family member). They could focus on any number of things, such as depression, anxiety, quality of life, hopelessness, suicidal ideation and so on.
2. **Ask Patrick to complete a non-standardised questionnaire:** This could focus on any area(s) that the therapist and Patrick feel are most important. For example he could give ratings out of ten for his happiness, activity levels, sleep or any other area of his life.
3. **Ask Patrick at the end of therapy whether the intervention was useful at a personal level for him:** This would be aimed at gaining more than just a yes/no answer. It could be based on a semi-structured interview, where information is gleaned on what it was about therapy that was useful or otherwise. This approach may even involve asking Patrick to complete a 'process measure', which is a form of questionnaire that looks more at what was useful about the act of therapy, rather than comparing before-and-after results on a questionnaire.
4. **Find out whether Patrick has resumed employment:** Patrick stopped working due to his emotional difficulties, so a good outcome of therapy could be that he feels able to go back to work again.

Any of the above could be suitable ways of evidencing the usefulness of therapy. Whichever is selected, it is important to remember that the choice of evidence is not value-free, it is influenced by factors such as underpinning philosophy, logistics, pragmatics, policies and protocols.

> Therapists should consider, implement and adapt techniques for capturing outcomes throughout therapy (before, during and after).

## Underpinning philosophy

In the introduction we discussed how the therapies fit alongside each other (remember we said they sit along a loose continuum from scientific through humanist, constructionist and constructivist to spiritual approaches). Because of this, it is important to remember that the roots and epistemology of each therapy have a big part to play in evidencing outcomes.

By way of example, cognitive behavioural therapy is very much engaged with the process of evidencing the efficacy of therapy through scientific research. This research has led to the development of reliable, well validated[1] questionnaires/ outcome measures. As a result, it has gained great credibility amongst wider society as a useful intervention for many different psychological problems.

By contrast, narrative therapy takes the view that this scientific approach is reductionist. 'Reductionism' simply means that people's experiences are reduced to an inadequate level, which fails to capture all of the factors that influence a person's experience. The vast majority of narrative therapists view outcomes as a change in the stories and words people use to describe their experiences. Consequently, the standardisation of outcome evidence is not particularly consistent with the philosophy.[2]

## Logistics

In an ideal world, we would know in advance of therapy exactly how we are going to evidence the utility of the intervention. In some cases, services have a set protocol (usually questionnaires) that they issue before and after therapy. There are even institutions set up to support this process (for example see www.coreims.co.uk). In this ideal world, therapy would start and finish as expected. Then the outcomes could be easily and quickly interpreted. On the other hand, in this utopian world people wouldn't ever encounter a level of distress that would cause them to seek therapy.

The reality is often that even with the best of intentions, the measures available cannot truly capture the full impact of therapy. All too frequently, popular tools are not suitable for some people to complete. People regularly drop out of therapy without warning, and certainly without completing the hoped-for outcome measures. Furthermore, services often have their own logistical (often cost-based) factors that influence how outcomes are assessed:

> There is a great need for cost-effectiveness showing how much improvement in mental health, at a population or individual level is achieved by the implementation of often complex measurement applications. (Trauer, 2010: 81)

However, we must also remember that the decisions made by services are not only influenced by cost but also by legislation, as well as personal decisions around resource allocation, all of which have a set of values/beliefs that underpin the decisions (see Figure 12.2).

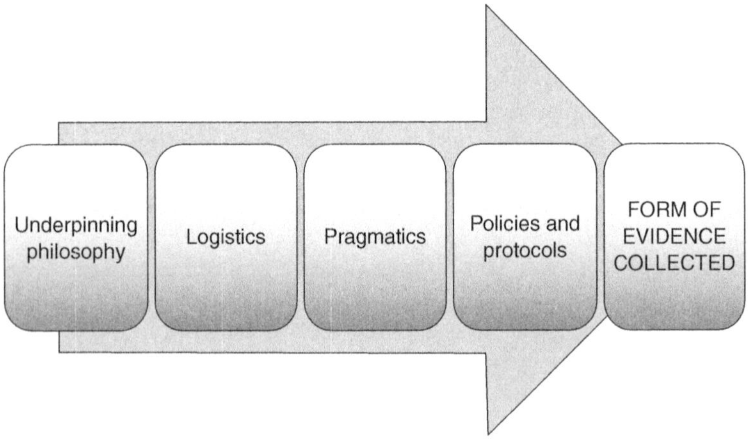


**Figure 12.2** The logistics of therapy

## Pragmatics

Let's begin our look at pragmatics, with the slightly controversial view that therapists have a bit of a default when it comes to the approaches they take. Some therapies just seem to sit better with us. Similarly, we may have preferences when it comes to outcome measurement, so personal preference has a part to play when it comes to selecting how to gather evidence. For example, we may prefer quantitative forms of evidence, which would naturally lead us more towards questionnaires. On the other hand, we may be more qualitatively minded, which may lead us more towards gathering information through interviews/discussions with people who access therapy. So long as we acknowledge, reflect upon and work with our own standpoint, it doesn't have to be a hindrance; in fact, it may help us to work better.

On a broader level, other factors that may influence our approach include, and are not limited to: the time available to dedicate to gathering information; the availability of tools that focus on the area pertinent to therapy; the ability levels of us as therapists, and the person accessing therapy; the desire to place as little demand on the person as possible in order to gather the necessary information.

Last, a statistic that should be interesting regardless of context and perspective. For example, an investigation that looked at publications which included outcome measures found that 1,430 outcome measures were used during the five-year period it examined, and of those 851 were used just once (Froyd et al., 1996). This suggests that a lot of outcome measures are developed which have no longevity. Outcome evaluation is of course an evolving area, but it is the responsibility of the clinician to ensure as best they can that however they evaluate outcomes, they attempt to do it in a meaningful manner.

## Policies and protocols

The responsibility for selecting what form of evidence to gather does not lie solely with the individual. The vast majority of therapists work in environments where they are bound to follow service policies. Outcome measurement in mental health has been referenced from at least as far back as the early twentieth century, and in the 1980s services as well as academics began focusing on quality of life as an outcome as well as expenditure (Trauer, 2010). There is little doubt that therapy can be effective; in fact, Corey (2009) reports that people who access therapy are up to 80 per cent better off than those who do not. However, the reality is that therapy and therapists as a resource have a cost, and every budget is finite. Services, commissioners, and indeed the general public want the best outcome for the least possible cost.

If we assume that part of why we are therapists is because we believe that therapy can be useful to people, then our challenge, regardless of our stage of development, is to show how and why our particular approach can be both useful and cost-effective (even if it is not readily quantifiable). The most common way of considering the evidence from outcome evaluation is to grade it according to a hierarchy ranging from well-designed randomised controlled trials (highest quality) to expert opinion based on clinical evidence. Therapies that present the most positive data, in the most respected form, are most likely to be supported (both theoretically and practically).

Therapeutic approaches that do not conform to this scientific approach run the risk of being marginalised. However, it's not all doom and gloom for therapies outside the positivist domain. It is

> If any of this really interests you, read some of the literature on evidence-based practice and practice-based evidence (e.g. Barkham, et al., 2010).

still possible to take part in the debate without conforming to the dominant perspective. There are many different forms of evidence, and many different ways to disseminate that evidence.

To conclude, the term 'outcomes' can mean different things to different people but it is essentially supposed to be a way of showing whether or not therapy has been useful. It is influenced by a range of factors, including what you and the person accessing therapy bring to the experience, how therapeutic your relationship is, what techniques you use, and many other factors that could take a lifetime to describe and are ever changing. Selecting how to capture that evidence is influenced by factors on an individual, system/service and societal level.

What you do with all of this information and where you go from here is up to you. Hopefully you'll explore at least some of it a bit more. Whether you are new to therapy or have been a therapist for many years, the decisions you make at every stage can influence not only what happens in therapy now, but also how the future of therapy is shaped.

## WHAT NEXT?

It is difficult to predict what the future holds for talking therapies, but hopefully they will continue to be recognised as useful tools for helping to reduce emotional distress. Outcome evidence is likely to be a key factor in therapies that gain momentum and standing in the coming years. The danger is that therapeutic methods may adapt to make capturing outcomes easier at the expense of losing focus on the person/people who are involved in the process (including the therapist).

There has been a trend recently towards manualised approaches and computer-based therapy. This may be due to these approaches being easier to standardise for research, or because they are cost-effective. We do not dismiss these approaches, in fact self-help interventions such as these can have quite an empowering role. For many people, they are also more readily available and accessible than direct therapy. However, it is important that these approaches are seen as an adjunct to direct contact with a therapist, not a replacement for that relationship. As the evidence from Lambert (1992) shows, losing that relationship could mean losing around 30 per cent of the potential outcome of therapy.

Therapy will always evolve. New therapies have developed in the last 20 years and more will be developed in the next 20 years. There seems to be a trend towards more integrative approaches that incorporate the 'best bits' from established models, some of which have been covered in this book (e.g. cognitive analytical therapy, dialectical behaviour therapy). It is likely that other integrative approaches will also develop; for example, we may see systemic cognitive behavioural therapy[3] or narrative-based mindfulness – who knows what will develop?

Some of the approaches discussed in this book (e.g. mindfulness) are already being incorporated into 'new-wave therapies'. The end of the CBT chapter introduces some of these approaches, with references for further reading. If *The Pocket Guide to Therapy* had been written 20–30 years ago, there may well have been greater reference to some of the approaches that were previously dominant (e.g. behavioural therapy) but have since been more widely subsumed into other therapies. Equally, if this book were re-written in 20 years' time, we would inevitably not see some of the current models included, in favour of newer models such as acceptance and commitment therapy and compassionate-focused therapies.

As technology and our understanding of the brain advances, it is also likely that we will see new therapies develop that have a leaning towards these fields. For example, in recent years the term 'neuropsychotherapy' has become more widely used, and attempts have been made to understand the neuroscience of psychotherapy (e.g. Cozolino, 2002). Perhaps this will lead to the birth of models such as psychodynamic neuropsychotherapy or trauma-focused neurocognitive therapy.

When new integrative therapies develop, there is often a response from classical therapists advocating that we do not lose sight of the purist approach of that particular therapy. The discussions around person-centred therapy offer an interesting example of this integrative versus purist debate. Both purist and integrative techniques have various pros and cons, and it's up to you as a developing therapist to see where you sit on the spectrum of approaches available in therapy. Our advice is to explore different models, see what feels best for you and the people you work with. Best of luck!

> It can be useful to read the PCT literature to get an idea of some of the arguments for and against each approach (see History section of Chapter 8).

## GLOSSARY

| | |
|---|---|
| Epistemology | Pilosophical understandings of what constitutes knowledge. |
| Generalisability | The ability of something (e.g. a questionnaire) to be applied in a range of different settings. |
| Holistic | An understanding of the different parts, which come together to create the whole. |
| Manualised | Therapy that follows a set pattern, using set techniques in a set format. This enables each aspect to be delivered in the same way each time, and presented in manual/textbook form. |

| | |
|---|---|
| Process measure | A tool for assessing what occurs during therapy. They give a good indication of how a person has experienced therapy, and what aspects were helpful or unhelpful about it. |
| Randomised controlled trial | An experiment where the participants are randomly allocated to receive one of a number of available approaches (e.g. therapy or medication). |
| Reductionist | A negative inference of scientific approaches, implying that they reduce experiences to a base level that fails to capture the complexity of influences on a person's experience. |
| Reliability | How consistent something (e.g. a questionnaire) is in capturing what it is supposed to capture, validity. |
| Standardised questionnaire | A questionnaire that has been researched by administering it to a lot of people. The results are statistically analysed to find out the result we would expect to see in any given population. |
| Validity | The level at which a conclusion accurately reflects what is actually happening in the real world. For example, if a person's results on a questionnaire looking at anxiety improve, are they actually less anxious than they used to be? |

## REFERENCES

Barkham, M., Hardy, G.E. and Mellor-Clark, J. (2010) *Developing and Delivering Practice-based Evidence: A Guide for the Psychological Therapies*. Chichester: Wiley-Blackwell.

Corey, G. (2009) *Theory and Practice of Counselling and Psychotherapy* (8th edn). Belmart, CA Wadsworth.

Cozolino, L. (2002) *The Neuroscience of Psychotherapy: Building and Rebuilding the Human Brain*. London: Norton.

Feltham, C. (2006) 'Counselling and psychotherapy in context', in C. Feltham and I. Horton (eds), *The SAGE Handbook of Counselling and Psychotherapy*. London: Sage.

Froyd, J.E., Lambert, M.J. and Froyd, J.D. (1996) 'A review of practices of psychotherapy outcome measurement', *Journal of Mental Health*, *5*, 11–16.

Lambert, M.J. (1992) 'Implications of outcome research for psychotherapy integration', in J.C. Norcross and M.R. Goldstein (eds), *Handbook of Psychotherapy Integration* (pp. 94–129). New York: Basic Books.

Lysaker, P. H., Lancaster, R. S. and Lysaker, J.T. (2003) 'Narrative transformation as an outcome in psychotherapy of psychosis', *Psychology and Psychotherapy*, *76*, 285–99.

Trauer, T. (2010) *Outcome Measurement in Mental Health: Theory and Practice*. Cambridge: Cambridge University Press.

## NOTES

1. Statistical terms showing the quality of the subject at hand, in this case an outcome measure.
2. For an exception to this perspective, see Lysaker et al. (2003).
3. Some CBT does involve the wider system as part of the 'environment' aspects.

# THE CHALLENGES

Every author in this book has qualified within the last three years, and so can remember what it's like to try to get to grips with a how-to-'do' therapy. Here's some thoughts on the challenges each model presented when writing about them.

## CHAPTER 2 MOTIVATIONAL INTERVIEWING

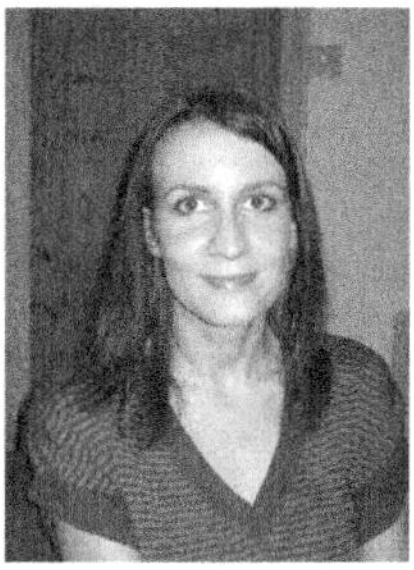

### Claire Robson

Whilst I longed for a brief and 'hands-on' introductory text during my own training, I found the process of describing MI in this way to be a real challenge. I felt that there was a huge risk of oversimplifying MI, and focusing too much on the techniques at the expense of the 'spirit'. It was tricky to provide the reader with a summary of the approach as a whole, whilst also bringing it to life and enabling the reader to come away with a sense of how it could be applied in day-to-day practice. Hopefully at least some of this has been achieved, and that it is clear how an MI style can be used in any situation in which there is some ambivalence to change a problem behaviour.

## CHAPTER 3 COGNITIVE BEHAVIOURAL THERAPY

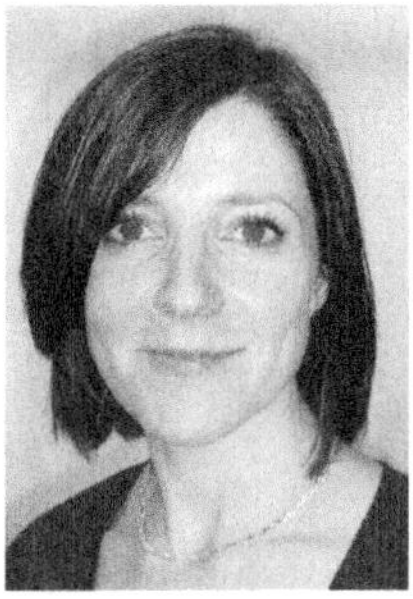

### Jane Toner

I wanted to present CBT as a credible form of therapy, not just a handful of 'techniques' and 'tools' that some people perceive (and promote) as CBT. I wanted to give priority to the therapeutic relationship within CBT, and emphasise the importance of a mutual and trusting relationship. I wanted to show how particular aspects of CBT can actually enhance that with many people. I wanted to write about skills that are often overlooked, particularly Socratic dialogue. I also wanted to mention that 'textbook' formulations can be used if they help, but that formulations have to be individualised and developed according to need. I believe that if people are taught CBT well, it can be adapted to most people's situation, but I also wanted to get the message over that CBT is not the 'be all and end all'. We can adapt our therapeutic approach in accordance with the person's needs, at that time, and CBT can be a very useful tool to have.

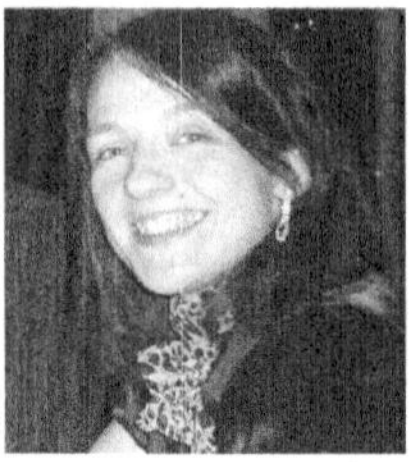

## CHAPTER 4
## COGNITIVE ANALYTIC THERAPY

### Sharon Twigg

My aim for this chapter was to break down the many misconceptions I have heard about the complexity of CAT therapy. However, trying to explain the CAT model using basic terminology and limited word space was no easy feat. It is a model that has a number of important parts that need explaining before you can understand how they fit together. The snag was trying to do this without falling into the trap of using too much CAT jargon or waffling over the word limit.

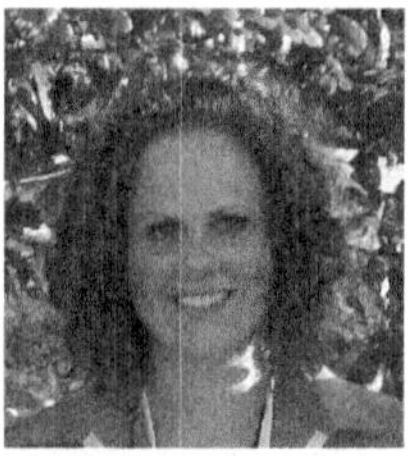

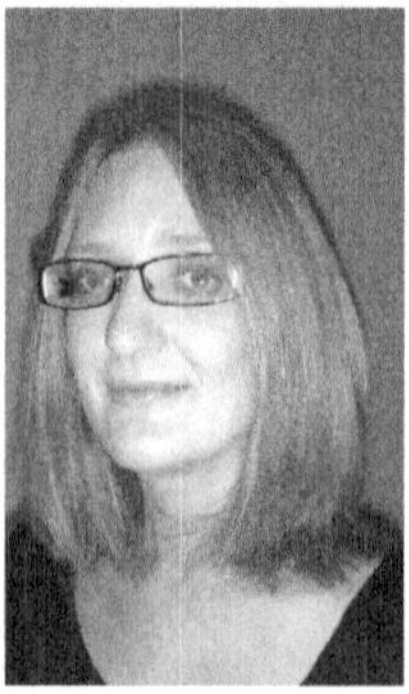

## CHAPTER 5
## PSYCHODYNAMIC THERAPY

### Amie Smith and Kara Garforth

There are so many models which fall under the umbrella of psychodynamic therapy. We tried to present concepts that are broadly shared by all these models, but we worried that we may be oversimplifying it at times. In terms of application, a big challenge is that there is no single set way of practising psychodynamic therapy. The model is process based, and so may feel less concrete than other models. For those new to practising the approach this may create a challenge, as you tend not to plan sessions and have to be flexible and responsive to the person, which can often create anxiety. Beginning to work with transference can be quite unnerving but really you have to do it and feel it, and then reflect on it. It is important that you are able to reflect on your part of the therapy process, which can really shake your confidence. It really helps to have good supervision to support you with this.

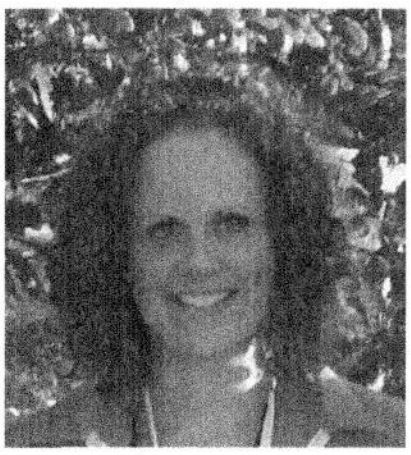

## CHAPTER 6
## SYSTEMIC THERAPIES

### Amie Smith and Stephen Weatherhead

Given the many schools, different approaches and ways of practising systemic therapy, we found it challenging to reach a consensus on which concepts to include. In systemic therapy the focus is on process and the bigger picture; as a therapist this can feel less concrete, more complex and at times perplexing. In the chapter, what we hope to have done is given you the overall concepts, and then offered techniques that could help you apply each concept (for example, to apply the concept of context you may use genograms). We hope that this brings the model to life a bit.

## CHAPTER 7
## NARRATIVE THERAPY

### Stephen Weatherhead

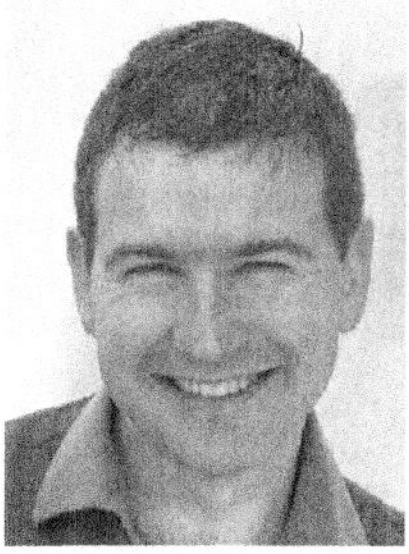

Narrative therapy is very closely linked to the philosophy on which it is built. This has led to many writers using language that feels unfamiliar, and a bit difficult to understand. It was important to me that this chapter explained the philosophy and practice of narrative therapy, but in an accessible way. Many of the better known texts in narrative therapy emphasise the work done in child and family settings, so I also wanted to show its applicability to a wide range of settings, regardless of age, context and other factors that people often think are outside of the remit of narrative therapy. All this was a challenge, but hopefully it makes sense.

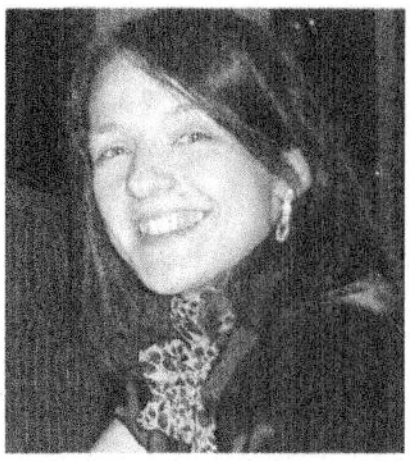

## CHAPTER 8
## PERSON-CENTRED THERAPY

### Sharon Twigg

This chapter was the more challenging of the two I wrote. Initially, the model seems straightforward to write about. However, I underestimated the complexity of trying to explain the different developmental stages of the selves and how outside factors affect these stages. I found myself drawing numerous diagrams in the hope of finding one that would explain the whole model, but ended up only confusing myself. Instead, I settled on 'bite-size' diagrams, which I hope are helpful to the reader.

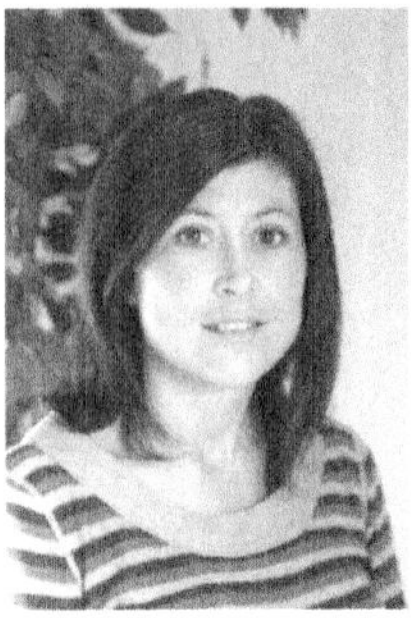

## CHAPTER 9 MINDFULNESS

### Katie Splevins

The main challenges when writing about mindfulness were in trying to explain a concept and way of being, which can really only be lived or experienced. Words are not really adequate to explain this and so trying to convey a sense of mindfulness in the broader sense was a challenge. Using words at times seemed to take something away from the concept, and I felt there was a risk I could oversimplify it (and while it is a very simple concept, the depth of the experience is vast). When practising the model it is a real challenge to commit enough time to your own development of mindfulness. For you to be a really effective mindfulness clinician it needs to be something you develop in your own life and work, which can require a lot of time and commitment.

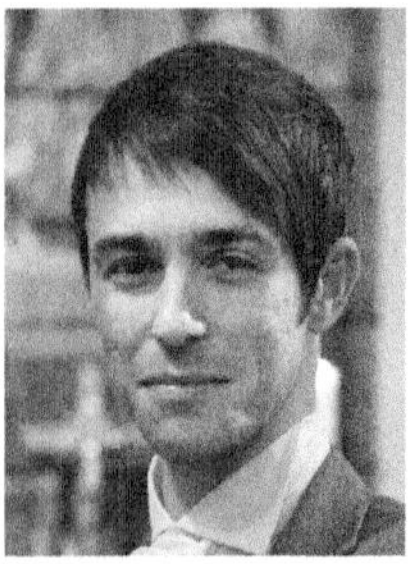

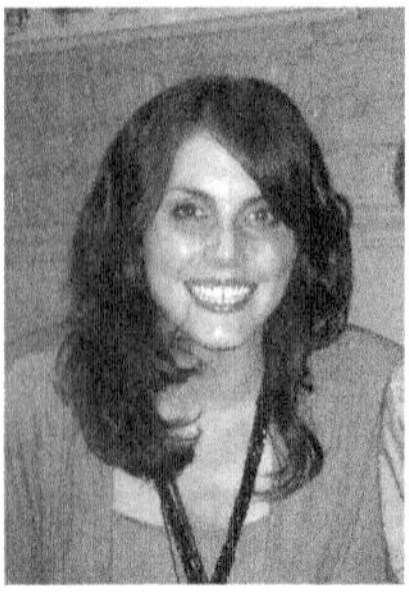

## CHAPTER 10 SOLUTION-FOCUSED BRIEF THERAPY

### Graeme Flaherty-Jones and Fiona Syme

SFBT is typically adapted to use the person's unique language and interests in therapy. While this is clearly a strength of the model, and one of the reasons we value the approach, it presented a challenge when trying to demonstrate how to apply the model in practice. As SFBT has such a non-mechanical approach, this may mean that professionals need to be more creative in how they evidence its efficacy. We have tried to show in the case examples how, regardless of the person's situation, their language and interests can be drawn on to guide interventions. True to SFBT, we hope this guides the reader in a non-directive manner on how to apply the model in therapy.

# CHAPTER 11
# DIALECTICAL BEHAVIOUR THERAPY

## Phillippa Calvert

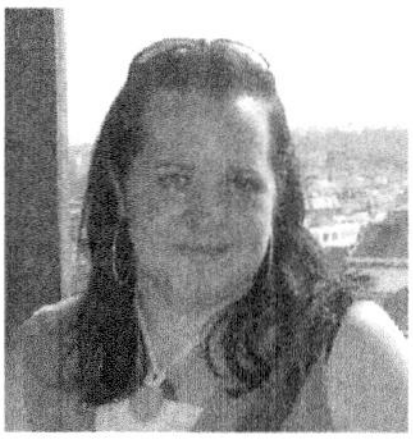

Respect, understanding and validation are explicitly built into DBT, with specific strategies to help the therapist retain this stance. I really like that DBT acknowledges that individuals with complex difficulties may need a therapeutic approach that aims to provide support and interventions in different ways. The biggest challenge was trying to summarise all the different elements and stages in DBT as the approach doesn't just include one-to-one therapy. Providing enough detail to allow the reader to learn about DBT and hopefully think about how to use the approaches in their own practice was difficult to say the least. I also wanted to demonstrate that the ideas could be used in a variety of settings. I only hope I have done it justice.

# INDEX